Seasons of Dance
The Story of Jamaican Dance Theatre

Seasons of Dance

The Story of Jamaican Dance Theatre

Photographed by Monica DaSilva

MACMILLAN
CARIBBEAN

Macmillan Education
Between Towns Road, Oxford OX4 3PP
A division of Macmillan Publishers Limited
Companies and representatives throughout the world

www.macmillan-caribbean.com

ISBN-13: 978-1-4050-7400-1
ISBN-10: 1-4050-7400-0

First published 2006

Designed by Susan Lee Quee
Typeset by Amanda Easter Design Ltd.

This book is dedicated to the dancers,
with special mention to Neville Black.

The cameras used are Minolta XD-7, X-300 and X-700; the lenses are fixed focal: 52mm, zoom: 28-70 mm and 70-210 mm.
I have not digitally changed the composition of the photographs in any way. All photographs were taken at Little Theatre,
Kingston, Jamaica unless otherwise stated.

The publishers have made every effort to trace all the dancers and choreographers involved in the photographs, but it
has not been possible to trace them all and they will be pleased to rectify any omissions or inaccuracies at the earliest
opportunity

Printed and bound in Thailand

2010 2009 2008 2007 2006
10 9 8 7 6 5 4 3 2 1

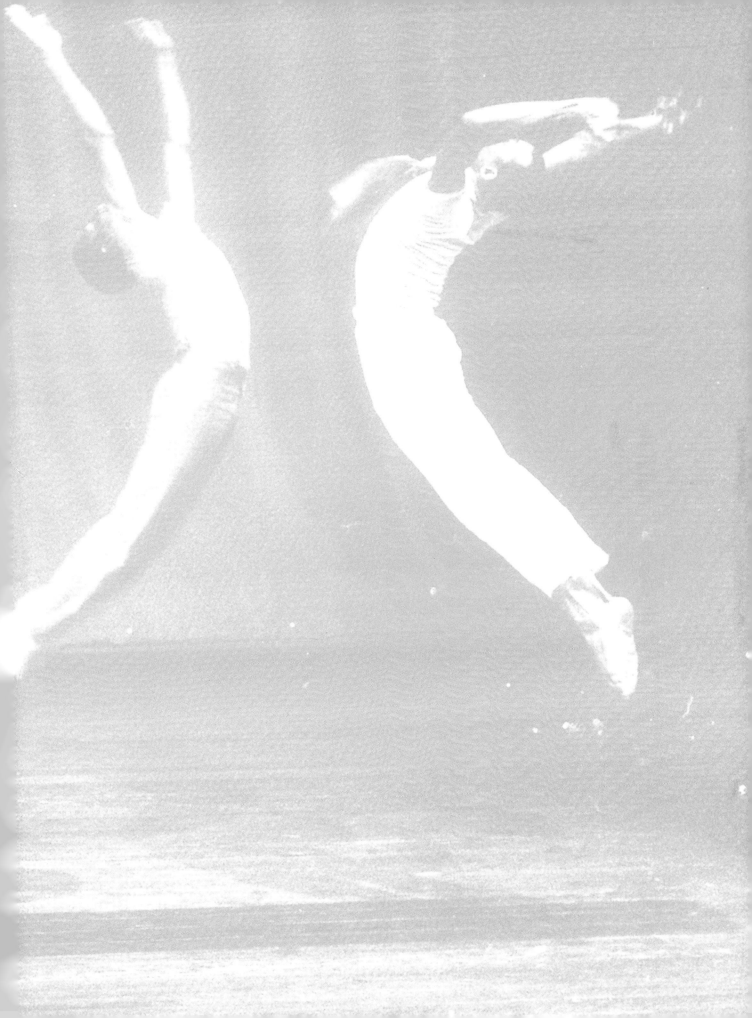

In loving memory of

Scott Matthew DaSilva

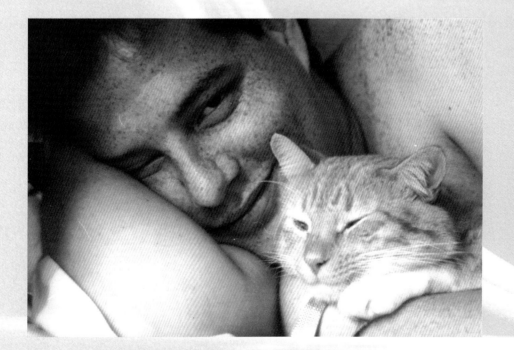

…upon the face of darkness

of the deep deep void

the great spirit danced

and the universe took form

the light

the waters too

living creatures

of every kind and species

plants flowers fruit and grain

appeared above the waters

and under the waters

then man and woman

the first of their kind

and it was good…

(adapted from the Bible)

Contents

Acknowledgements

The author and publisher would like to thank the Movements Dance Company, the School of Dance, L'Acadco, The Company Dance Theatre, The Stella Maris Dance Ensemble, The National Dance Theatre Company and all their artistic directors, for their permission to use these photographs of their dances and dancers, and for their many kind contributions to this book.

We are also grateful to: Easton Lee (for his poem used throughout this book); Carole Orane Andrade, Patrick Johnson, MoniKa Lawrence, Staci-Lee Hassan-Fowles for their photo editing; Photo Express, Ink Studios and Amalgamated (Distributors) Ltd (who printed the photographs); all the dancers, choreographers, singers, musicians, teachers, and costume, set and lighting designers who have worked on the dances featured in this book.

Preface

I was once asked what I wanted to communicate with this book. I answered that I'd like to show the beauty and dexterity of the human body, but it's much more than that. When a dancer steps on to that stage, he/she is putting to use years of training and hundreds of hours of rehearsals to do justice to the choreographer's idea for any given dance. My job was to capture, in a split second, all the emotions that the body – from head to toe – is portraying.

All theatre is in the world of make-believe and dance is an integral part of that world. The camera is there to hold the moment forever: be it tenderness, conflict, love, hate or laughter, and catch an illusion of that dance.

I have been very fortunate to have been into so many dance companies and to have witnessed their growth and development. I have only worked with six companies, but there are many more now, and all showing the diversity of the dance and the culture of Jamaica.

I would like to thank the artistic directors for their vision, the choreographers for their imagination, and finally, the dancers – whether they're in this book or not – for their talent. I hope that they will be pleased with how I've portrayed them. This book is for the dancers, of the dancers and to the dancers.

Monica DaSilva

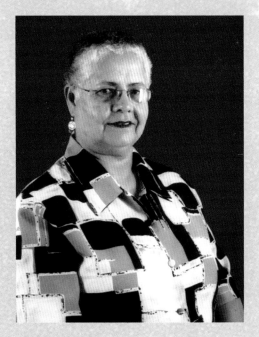

Foreword

The story of Jamaican dance-theatre precedes August 1962, when The National Dance Theatre Company (NDTC) flowered into existence at the time of Jamaica's Independence. In the 1950s and early 1960s, Jamaican dance-theatre started to assume ideal, form and purpose in a movement spearheaded by Ivy Baxter. Her group flourished in these years and spawned many founding directors and members of the NDTC. These people, along with others, have been the NDTC's flagship entity for over four decades and steered Jamaican dance-theatre to international acclaim. It is important to state that Jamaican dance's ancestral legacy also comes from its slave forebears, who used dance and music as strategies for survival in their lives of service.

Monica DaSilva's photographic essay *Seasons of Dance*, is inspired not only by the NDTC, but also by four other dance ensembles which have sprung up since the 1980s. In 1976, the Jamaica School of Dance was formed by dancer-choreographers Sheila Barnett, Barbara Requa and Bert Rose, in collaboration with the NDTC as a feeder source for performance of excellence, to promote dance education and research and to foster community outreach. In 1981, the Movements Dance Company emerged, and is now directed by Monica Campbell (who, with three other co-founders, was a former collaborator with Eddy Thomas, a founding director of the NDTC, in his short-lived Jamaican Dance Company). In 1983, the L'Acadco ensemble mounted its first Jamaican Season under the direction of L'Antoinette Stines, whose ancestral roots in Jamaican dance go back to her mentor Alma Mock Yen in the Harbour View Community Workshop. Alma Mock Yen was a moving spirit and principal with the Ivy Baxter Creative Dance Group in the 1950s. Coming much later was The Company Dance Theatre under the artistic direction of Tony Wilson, an NDTC alumnus and budding choreographer. More recently, MoniKa Lawrence (herself an NDTC alumna and principal as well as a choreographer) formed The Stella Maris Dance Ensemble of young adults.

Her work benefited from the opportunity to compete and win medals in annual festivals organised by the Jamaica Cultural Development Commission (JCDC), whose community work in dance received its initial impetus in 1963 from both the NDTC's Joyce Campbell and one of its artistic co-directors.

All these post-1980s dance ensembles now flourish on their own. Each moulds a novel orientation in Jamaican dance-theatre and expands the audience(s) for theatre-dance through annual Seasons of Dance, as well as television and other performances – thus releasing the art from its pre-Independence entrapment as a cultural minority indulgence based on colour, class and social snobbery.

The Ivy Baxter Group was not alone in keeping Jamaican dance alive. The European classical ballet studios, with links to the Royal Academy of Dance in the UK (and marginally to Russian and Canadian ballet training traditions), fed into The National Dance Theatre Company a number of well-trained pupils. These former pupils and their successors have contributed tremendous texture, diversity, versatility, creative tension, and dynamism in this cross-fertilisation process – the historical and existential life of Jamaica has dictated this, and still does. It is therefore easy to locate the NDTC and all these other groups in their quest for their own unique 'voices' within the mission/vision of the aesthetic, which reflects the inner logic and consistency of a culturally diverse Jamaica and the wider Caribbean.

All these dance ensembles turn naturally to traditional lore and contemporary popular idioms for inspiration – from ancestral pocomania and kumina, through myal and dinkimini, to latter-day reggae and dance-hall. The African presence here suggests itself in works from *African Scenario* (1962) to *Dance Jallof* (in the 1990s). The dance dramas depict specifically Caribbean and universal themes, as well as works exploring pure movement.

The shapes of the movements in all of these dance ensembles also contribute to the story of Jamaican dance and dance-theatre. Contact with the Earth is often contrasted with the litheness of airborne jumps and leaps. The moulded character of a three-dimensional form (suggesting voluptuousness) is juxtaposed with stretched and tensile reach in cantilevered arabesques in conquest of space. The isolation of pelvis and ribcage, often to counterpoint rhythm, is framed by fluid arms, undulating and carried in progression, upright or horizontal, flat-backed, to the floor.

Jamaica's dance theatre has attracted scene painters, sculptors, costume designers and photographers of the ilk of Monica DaSilva, Maria LaYacona, Owen Minott, Denis Valentine and others. Painters and sculptors, costume designers and foreign devotees attend the annual dance summer schools now run by the Jamaica School of Dance (a division of the Edna Manley College for Visual and Performing Arts), continuing a long established tradition by the University of the West Indies at Mona. These summer schools have attracted Caribbean dance artists as their teachers, such as Lavinia Williams, Leon Destine and Jean-Guy Saintus of Haiti, Beryl McBurnie of Trinidad, and Eduardo Rivero of Cuba – and their mentees have come to serve both the NDTC and Movements Dance Company as dancers. Modern dance teachers have also come from the USA, such as Neville Black (Jamaican born), Lew Smith, and John Jones, and more recently, Kariamu Asante of Temple University (who specialises in African dance).

The music of Europe, Latin America and the United States, as well as of Africa south of the Sahara, have all informed the on-going experimentation and exploration in Jamaican dance theatre – so have the compositions of Jamaican musicians Oswald Russell, Marjorie Whylie, Peter Ashbourne, and Grub Cooper (who have all written specifically for dance works performed by at least two of the dance companies).

It is this story of commitment to artistic integrity, sustained application and concentrated work among a motley crew of dancers, singers, and musicians – the vast majority of whom are still unpaid but dedicated performing volunteers, teachers, critics, fine artists, and costume and lighting designers – that has made Monica DaSilva's photographic essay such a rewarding and visually exciting document of Jamaican poetry in motion.

Rex Nettleford

Professor the Hon Rex Nettleford is Vice Chancellor Emeritus of the University of the West Indies. He is a founder, artistic director and principal choreographer of The National Dance Theatre Company of Jamaica, and a recently-appointed ambassador at large for Jamaica. Among his many published works are Dance Jamaica – Cultural Definitions and Artistic Discovery *(Grove Press, N.Y. 1985) and* Roots and Rhythms *(Andre Deutsch, London 1969).*

What makes a great dance photograph?

The answer varies according to the needs of the viewer.

To the dance artist, it is the need to capture for posterity, the beauty and form of the performer as he/she executes a miraculous series of dance movements – the outcome of years of hard work and training. To the choreographer, it is a means of capturing still shots which can document his/her work of art. To the dance teacher, the photograph is a record of the level of accomplishment achieved by the students – an individual dancer or a group of dancers – and perhaps a means of archival documentation for the studio or school. To the parent of the young dancer, it is a cherished memory of the early days and the many trips made transporting the child to classes and performances.

Dance Art is ephemeral, transient – the creation of visual pictures that remain with the viewer for fleeting moments only to disappear…until the next performance. It leaves nothing of permanence except the fragments of paper carefully pasted in an album for future viewing.

Robert Greskovic, a critic of dance photography, sees them as 'frozen fragments of first-hand fleeting experiences best appreciated after viewing the performance itself'. Another dance critic describes photographs of dance as 'amoeba-shaped blobs…isolated in the camera field (as objects) hanging in a void, in nowhere'. He decries the inability of photographs to capture the rhythm and motion of dance. Such criticisms are extreme, perhaps reflecting the opinions of perfectionists. William A Ewing, acclaimed dance photographer, suggests that, at its best, dance photography should 'take on an artistic life of its own, as an independent medium subject to its own laws'.

In my opinion, the dance photograph is an important element of the dance art and serves all the needs stated above. A great dance photograph must be judged on the basis of the need, and the ability to supply this need (whether achieved by a professional photographer or an inexperienced viewer). The great dance photograph should not be posed for; it should emerge from the performance, thus reflecting the rhythm and motion of the dance.

Ultimately, it is clear that dance photography cannot be successfully achieved without expending a great deal of time and effort. Whether taken by the amateur or the professional, the dancer(s) has to be viewed and observed in the space for a number of times in order to capture the high point of each action – the fully extended body in flight; the exquisitely poised arabesque held for a breath before moving on to the next step; the opening statement or climax which carries the idea of the dance. This is dance photography at its most exciting level.

Monica DaSilva brings to dance photography a wealth of experience honed on over more than twenty years of practice. I am confident that her book, *Seasons of Dance: The Story of Jamaican Dance Theatre*, will serve the needs of all the companies and groups with whom she has worked: the performers, the teachers and the choreographers, and for the hard working parents there will be treasured memories of the early years.

Through her collection of photographs, Monica DaSilva will disclose the ethos of Jamaican dance – its rich cultural roots, its unique style – and possibly offer the viewer some insights into the development of theatre dance over the last twenty years. Somewhere on the journey we will recognise many, many great dance photographs: works of art, to be shared and appreciated by all who view this book, amateurs and professionals alike. ENJOY!

Barbara Requa

Former Dean of the Edna Manley
College for Visual and Performing Arts

Power, Passion and line:

Monica DaSilva, the accidental photographer

An eye and a connection to the unpredictable rhythm of disparate bodies on stage… An ability to capture, shape and refine movements as photographs… A twenty-year love affair with lens, line and light… That's what it took to capture what is an inimitable collection, a heritage of the world of Jamaican performance dance. All that has been the journey of Monica DaSilva, the accidental photographer.

Reputed as a modest photographer who has an incredible eye for grace and precision, always seeming to catch the near perfection dancer-expressions and performance themes, no other has visually documented the seasons of all major professional dance companies in Jamaica. No other has defined the art of dance using photography as Monica DaSilva has.

She has covered the seasons of The National Dance Theatre Company (NDTC), L'Acadco, Movements Dance Company, The Company Dance Theatre, and The Stella Maris Dance Ensemble among others. She has recorded slips, lifts and dips, has watched experimental work grow into iconic pieces, recites dance technical terms with equal ease as photography jargon, dates of performances and the names of dancers.

Monica DaSilva first picked up her camera to take family photos, but her instinctual, self-taught passion for films, their moving images and the stories they tell, later led to her passion for shooting the performing arts. From arts and culture festivals, plays, stage and television productions, arts and culture celebrities, she has been busy using what her late son Scott called her third eye. 'I use my camera like a video camera with it always up to my eyes…following the dancers…and what I find exciting is when you manage to capture something that even another photographer coming along will not get…' And now after a wild twenty-year ride, Monica DaSilva has wallowed in the creative yet sometimes painfully tedious task of choosing from thousands of photographs.

Her book *Seasons of Dance: The Story of Jamaican Dance Theatre* is a tribute to her late son Scott DaSilva, who was often her main cheerleader along the way. 'It's been twenty years…and I did not expect it…the body of work that I have and no one else has…wasn't something I was looking for…but simply progressively happened…'

What Monica DaSilva wants is for readers of this book to come away with 'a sense of the beauty of the human body and what the human body can do… I'd like to think that I've enhanced that as best I could. I'd like readers to say 'Wow…how did they do that? How did the dancers get into a position like that?' And for the dancers to feel great about how I've captured them.'

Monica DaSilva has won awards for her photography in the Jamaica Cultural Development Commission's (JCDC) Photographic National Competition. She has been a judge for the Jamaica JCDC Festival Photo Competition. Her 1984 Photo Exhibition was reviewed by the journalist Archie Lindo who said in part '… she has used her camera to create new methods of approach … of concept … another strength … is her marvellous way of using light … in her portraits. An artist with a camera, as good as they make … who will go on to great achievement in the not-to-distant future.'

Monica DaSilva's work has been printed in over 20 different publications in Jamaica, including the *Best of Skywritings*, Evon Blake's *Beautiful Jamaica* and *Bob Marley – Reggae King of the World*. Others are: *Jamaica By Night, Lifestyle Mag, Skywritings, The Gleaner, The Daily News, Jamaica Journal, Jamaica Pictorial, JCDC 25th Anniversary Publication, Pure Class, The Jamaica Record, The Weekend Star,* and *Dancescape.*

Ingrid Riley

Entrepreneur, Writer, Poet

Movements Dance Company

Movements Dance Company

In 1981, four dancers embraced a vision of their art form defined by innovation, versatility and an appreciation for their country's culture and heritage. Out of this vision, the Movements Dance Company of Jamaica was launched in March 1981. In developing this company, co-founders Monica Campbell, Pat Grant-Goshop, Michelle Tappin-Lee and Denise Desnoes conceived an institution that would centre on the collective effort of its members and make a tangible contribution to the development of dance in their island nation.

The Movements Dance Company has evolved into one of the country's most dynamic and versatile companies; recognised for its fresh approach to modern contemporary dance with a distinctly Jamaican flavour. It has become one of the foremost players in Jamaican performing arts, and a driving force behind its standards and development. With the infinite inspiration and meticulous eye of its artistic director Monica Campbell, the company's performances are an experience of vibrant interpretations set against a tapestry of diverse musical compositions, ranging from the classics to the rhythms of the Caribbean, and always with the reggae vibrations of Jamaica.

The company's repertoire includes works by Monica Campbell, members of the company and several distinguished local and overseas artistes. Among these artistes are Jackie Guy, a founding tutor and choreographer who now resides in the United Kingdom, and the late great Neville Black, another Jamaican tutor and choreographer, whose impact on the company's performance vocabulary has been significant.

Commitment is the cornerstone of the Movements Dance Company, which has maintained the highest standards of the art form despite the full-time professional and personal obligations of its members. A management committee including volunteers from the business and professional sectors sets the company's broad policy, co-ordinates its annual schedule of activities and organises fundraisers. The company's schedule of local performances climaxes each year with an annual Season of Dance in November. Overseas performances have taken the Movements Dance Company to the United Kingdom, the United States of America, Canada and the Caribbean.

Monica Campbell, Artistic Director

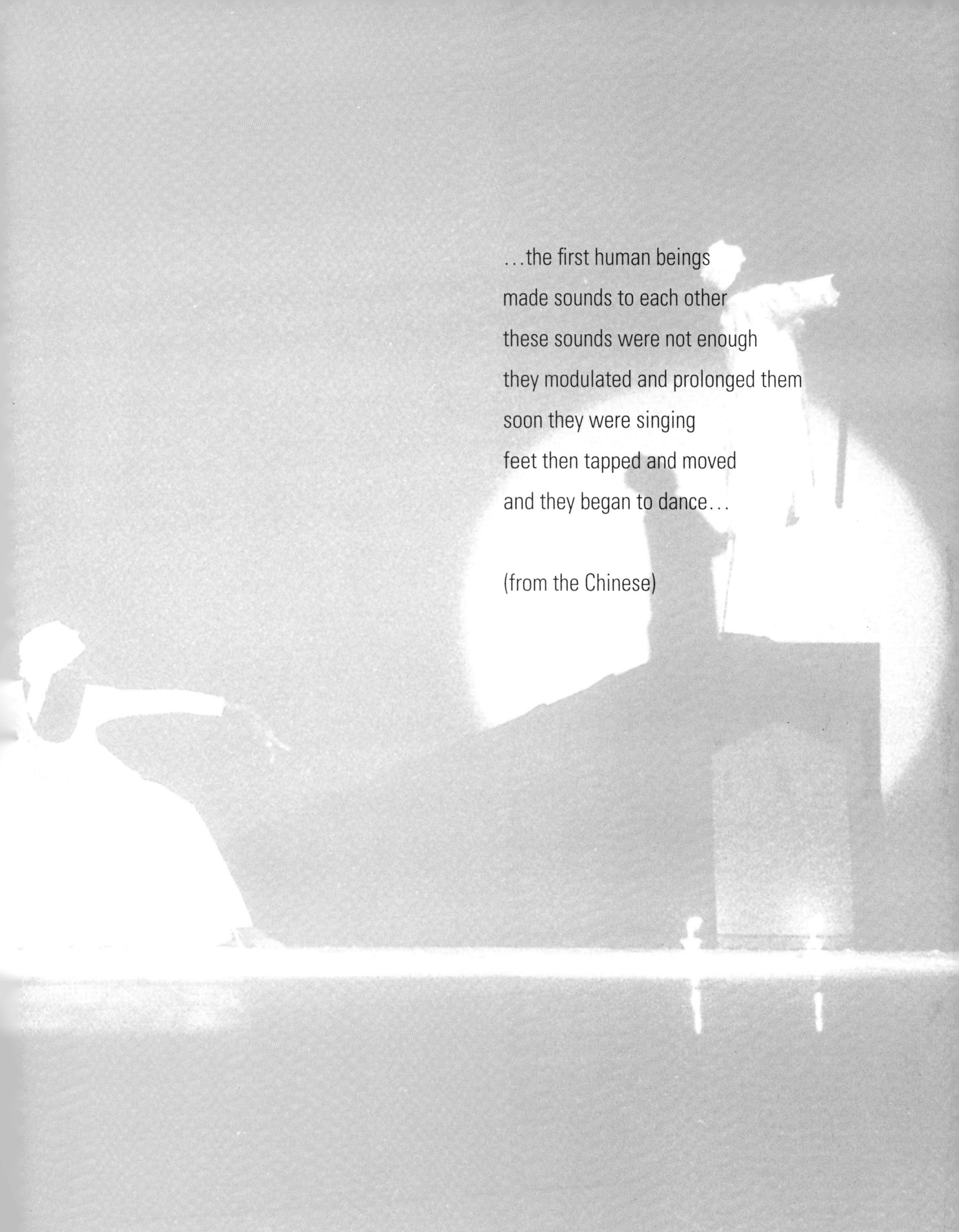

…the first human beings

made sounds to each other

these sounds were not enough

they modulated and prolonged them

soon they were singing

feet then tapped and moved

and they began to dance…

(from the Chinese)

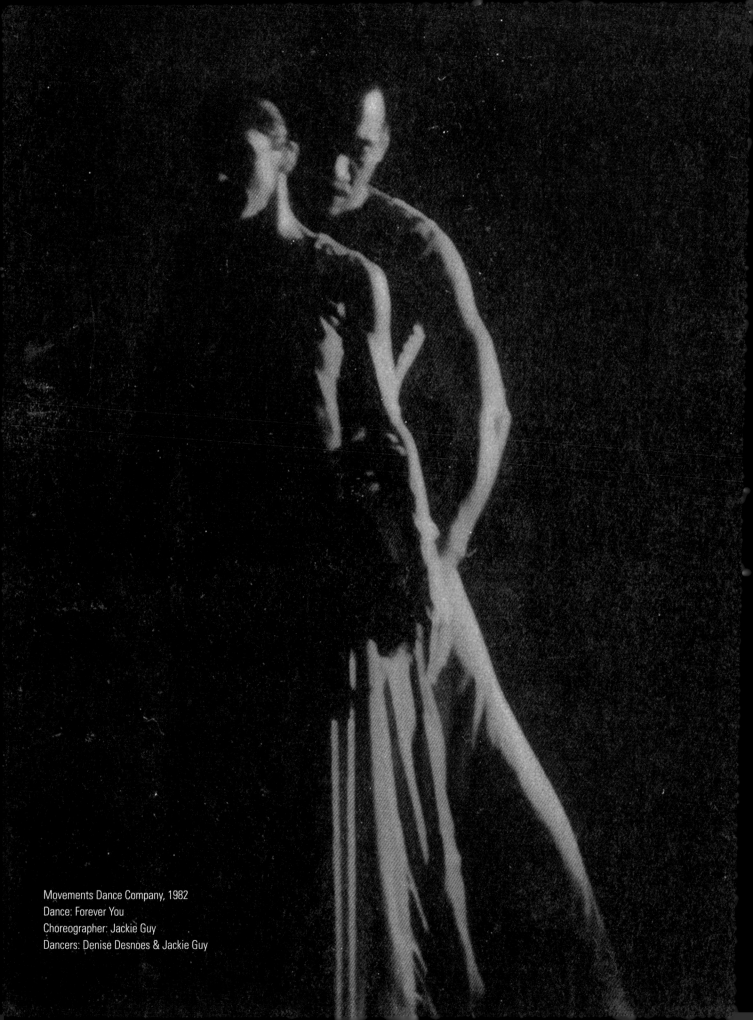

Movements Dance Company, 1982
Dance: Forever You
Choreographer: Jackie Guy
Dancers: Denise Desnoes & Jackie Guy

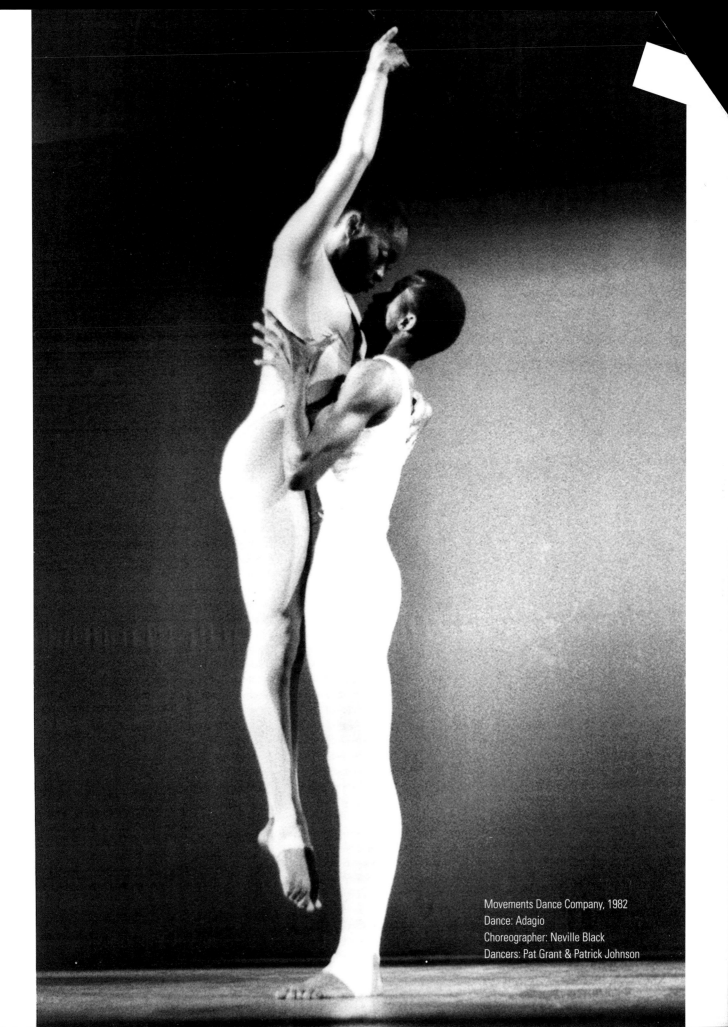

Movements Dance Company, 1982
Dance: Adagio
Choreographer: Neville Black
Dancers: Pat Grant & Patrick Johnson

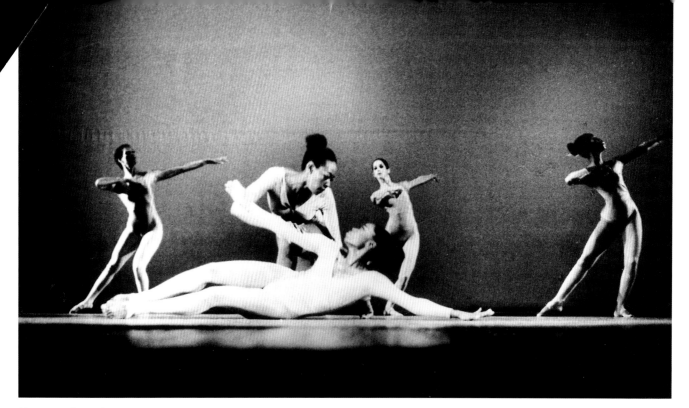

Movements Dance Company, 1982
Dance: Adagio
Choreographer: Neville Black
Dancers: Michelle Tappin-Lee, Paulette Cousins, Pat Grant,
Denise Desnoes & Terry Robinson

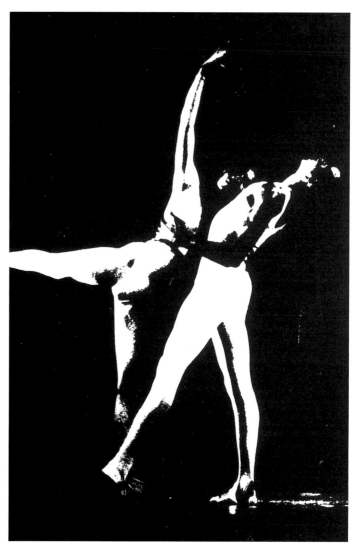

Movements Dance Company, 1982
Dance: Adagio
Choreographer: Neville Black
Dancers: Pat Grant & Patrick Johnson

Movements Dance Company, 1983
Dance: Bridges
Choreographer: Monica Campbell
Dancers: Michelle Tappin-Lee & Carol Levy

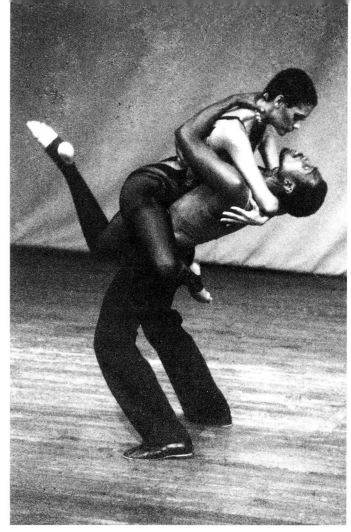

Movements Dance Company, 1982
Dance: Forever You
Choreographer: Jackie Guy
Dancers: Jackie Guy & Denise Desnoes

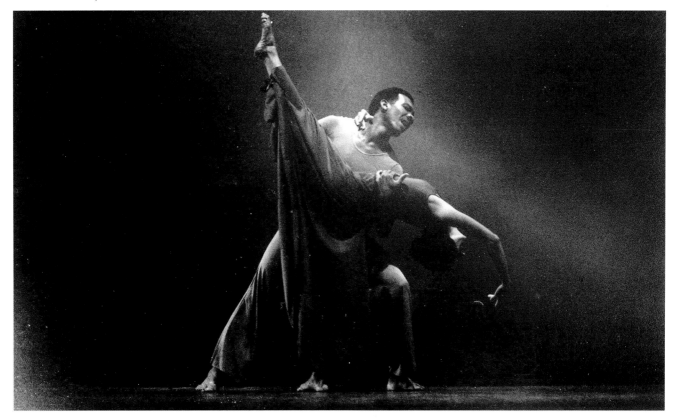

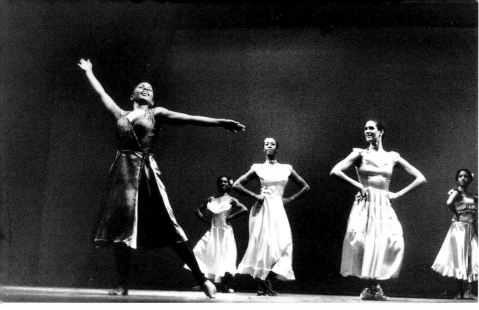

Movements Dance Company, 1983
Dance: Bridges
Choreographer: Monica Campbell
Dancers: Laurie-Ann Taylor, Hillary Coley, Paulette
Cousins, Michelle Tappin-Lee & Judith Henriques

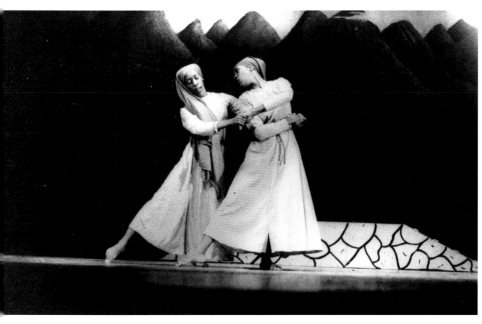

Movements Dance Company, 1983
Dance: Ruth
Choreographer: Jackie Guy
Dancers: Hillary Coley & Paulette Cousins

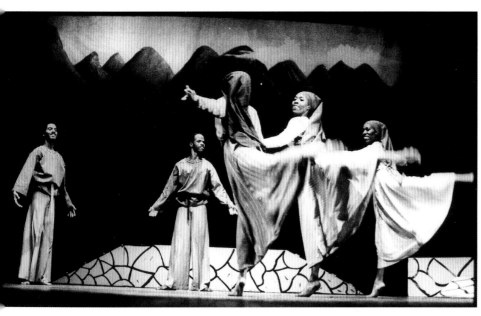

Movements Dance Company, 1983
Dance: Ruth
Choreographer: Jackie Guy
Dancers: Wayne Campbell, Mark Ramsey, Judith
Henriques, Paulette Cousins & Hillary Coley

…and in the garden

the serpent danced

coiling around the sinful tree

the man and the woman

joined in the dance

their children too

David the king,

Ruth and Miriam

Aaron, Salome

And the prophets of Baal…

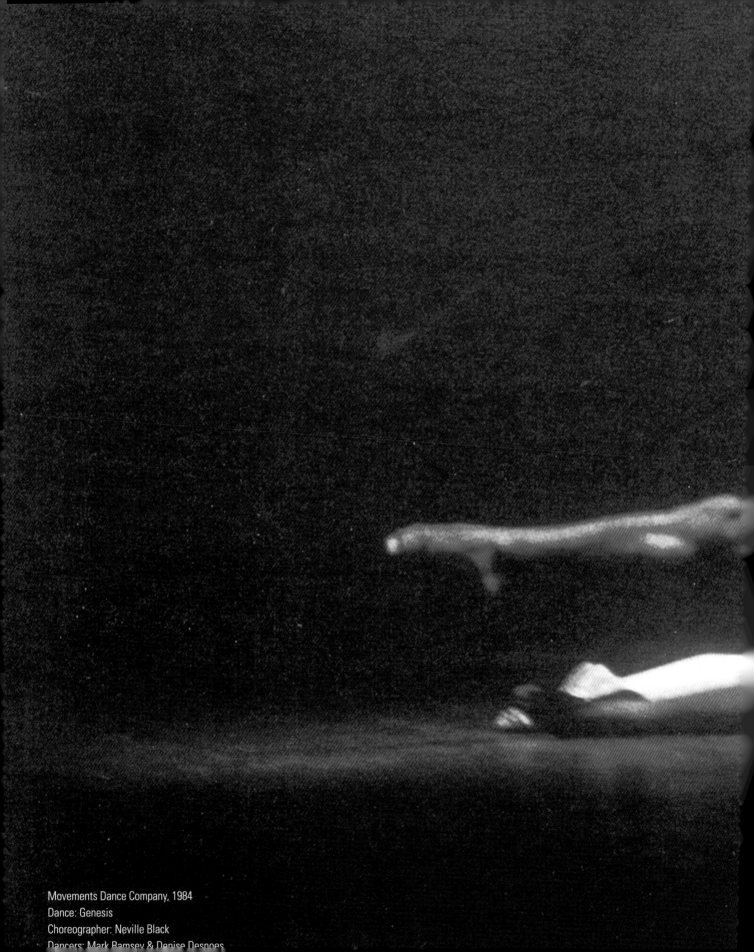

Movements Dance Company, 1984
Dance: Genesis
Choreographer: Neville Black
Dancers: Mark Ramsey & Denise Despoes

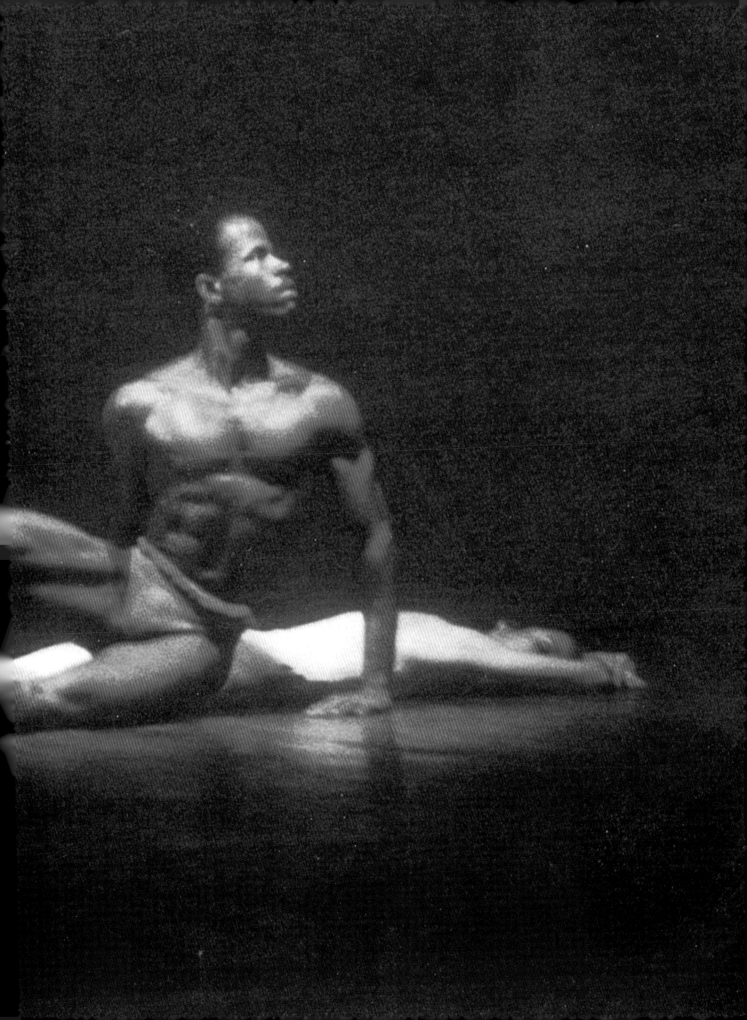

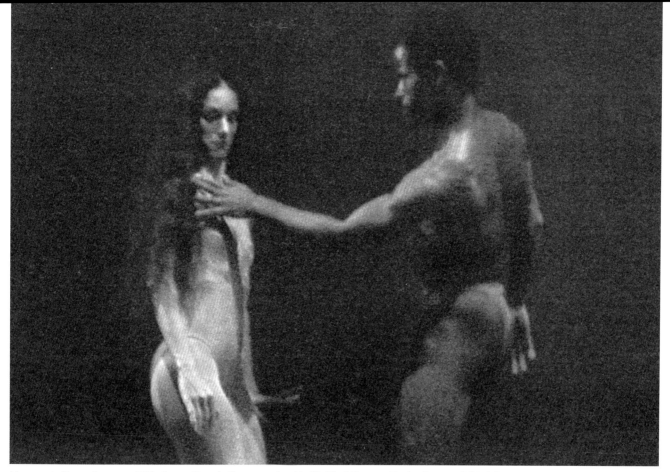

Movements Dance Company, 1984 Dance: Genesis Choreographer: Neville Black Dancers: Denise Desnoes & Mark Ramsey

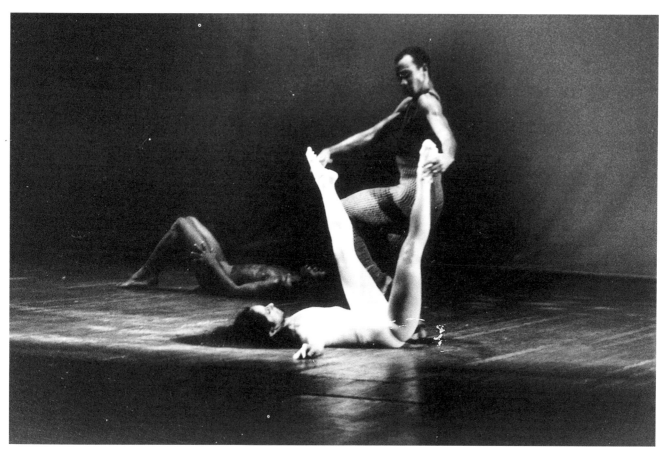

Movements Dance Company, 1984 Dance: Genesis Choreographer: Neville Black Dancers: Mark Ramsey, Denise Desnoes & Patrick Johnson

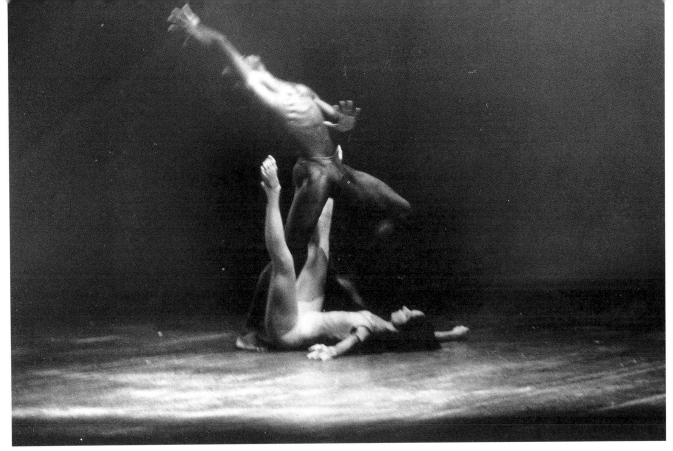

Movements Dance Company, 1984 Dance: Genesis Choreographer: Neville Black Dancers: Mark Ramsey & Denise Desnoes

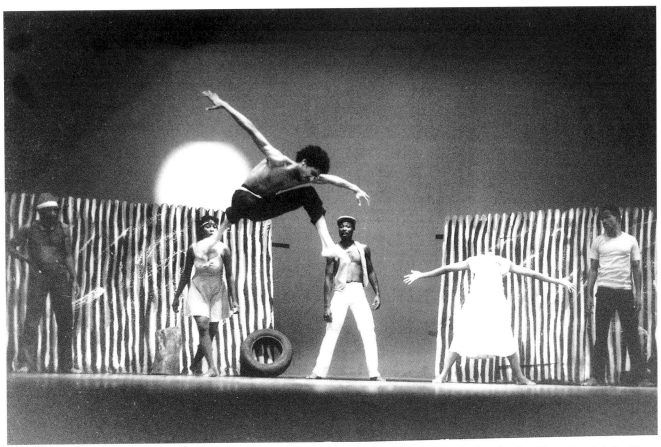

Movements Dance Company, 1984 Dance: Pressure Choreographer: Monica Campbell Dancers: Jackie Guy, Paulette Cousins, Wayne Campbell, Carol Levy, Hillary Coley & Mark Ramsey

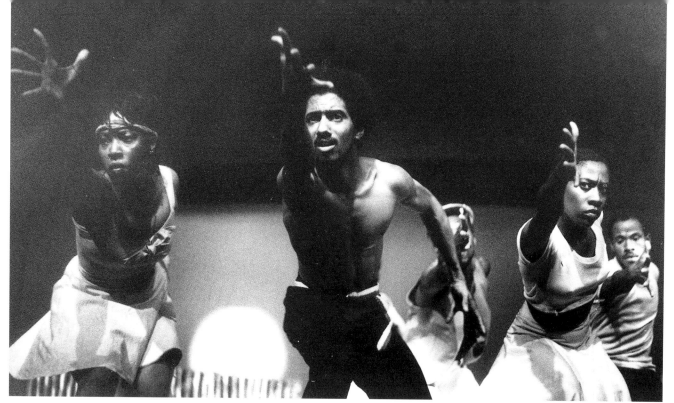

Movements Dance Company, 1984 Dance: Pressure Choreographer: Monica Campbell Dancers: Paulette Cousins, Wayne Campbell, Carol Levy, Hillary Coley & Mark Ramsey

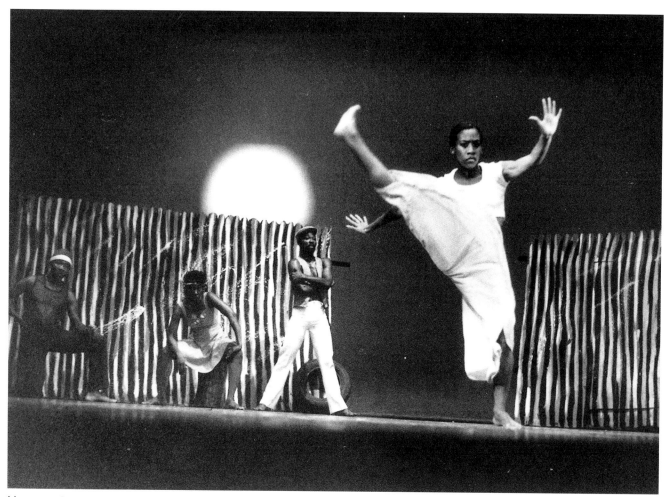

Movements Dance Company, 1984 Dance: Pressure Choreographer: Monica Campbell Dancers: Jackie Guy, Paulette Cousins, Carol Levy & Hillary Coley

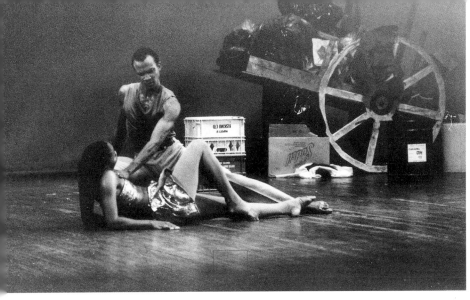

Movements Dance Company, 1984
Dance: Dinah's Song
Choreographer: Keith Noel
Dancers: Pat Grant & Patrick Johnson

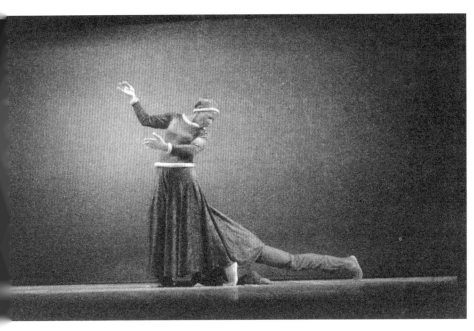

Movements Dance Company, 1984
Dance: Four Ambiguous Dances
Choreographer: Neville Black
Dancers: Monica Campbell & Patrick Johnson

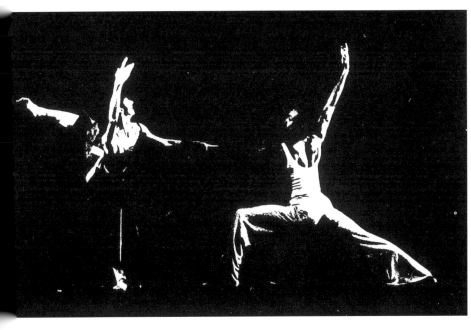

Movements Dance Company, 1985
Dance: Tribute to Bach
Choreographer: Neville Black
Dancers: Denise Desnoes & Patrick Johnson

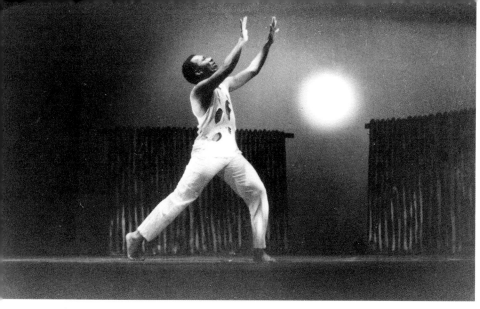

Movements Dance Company, 1985
Dance: Pressure
Choreographer: Monica Campbell
Dancer: Jackie Guy

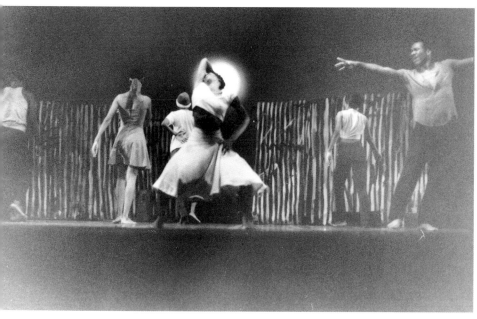

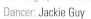

Movements Dance Company, 1985
Dance: Pressure
Choreographer: Monica Campbell
Dancers: Nigel Hinds, Michelle Tappin-Lee, Marcia
McKenzie, Hillary Coley, Sharon Tai & Jackie Guy

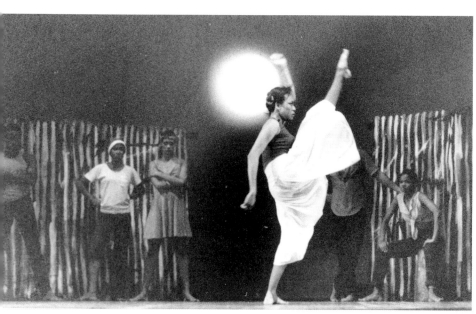

Movements Dance Company, 1985
Dance: Pressure
Choreographer: Monica Campbell
Dancers: Nigel Hinds, Pat Grant, Michelle Tappin-Lee,
Sharon Tai & Jackie Rose

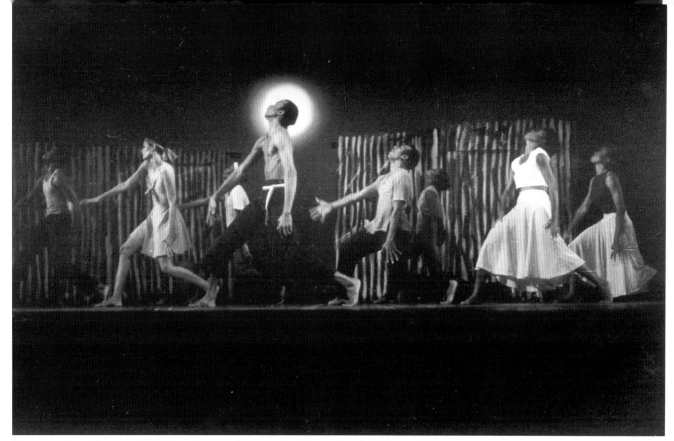

Movements Dance Company, 1985 Dance: Pressure Choreographer: Monica Campbell Dancers: The Company

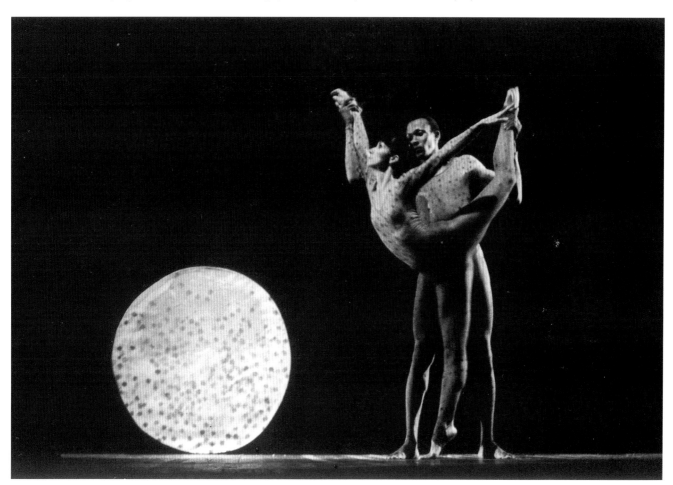

Movements Dance Company, 1985 Dance: Mitosis Choreographer: Jackie Guy Dancers: Denise Desnoes & Patrick Johnson

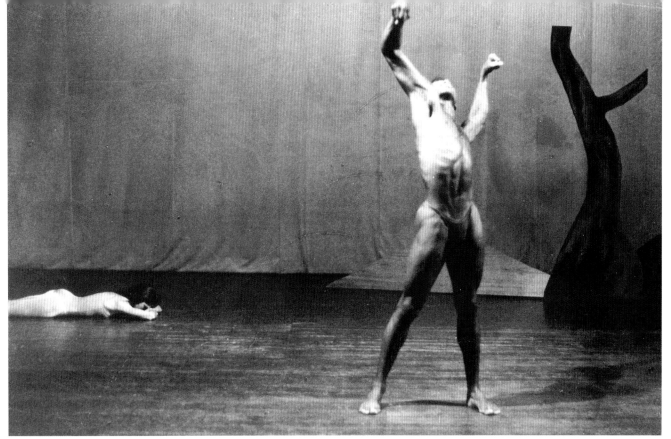

Movements Dance Company, 1986 Dance: Genesis Choreographer: Neville Black Dancers: Denise Desnoes & Garth Sinclair

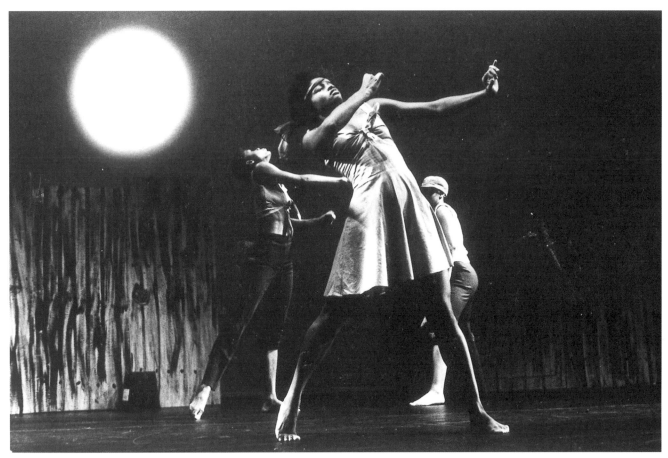

Movements Dance Company, 1986 Dance: Pressure Choreographer: Monica Campbell Dancers: Marcia McKenzie, Jackie Rose & Dawn Wilson
(Shaw Theatre, London)

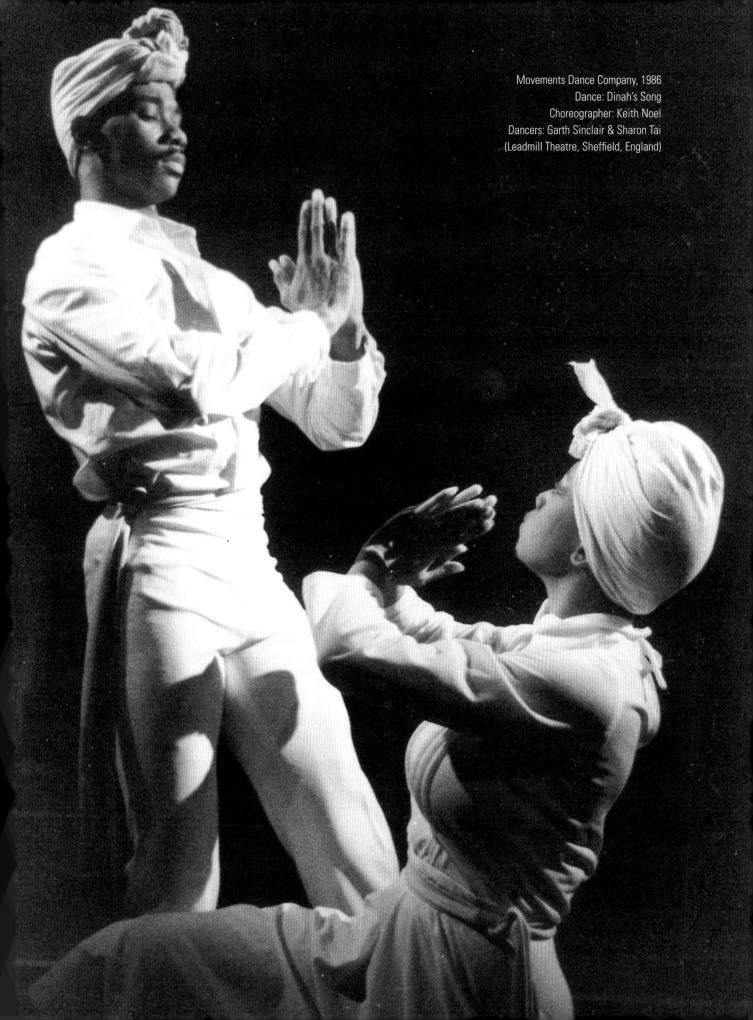

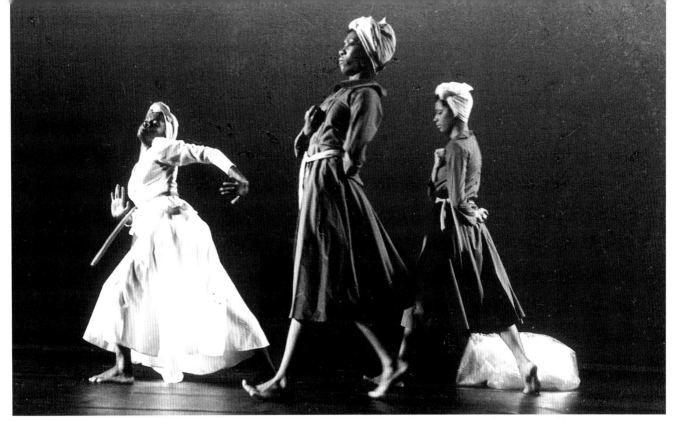

Movements Dance Company, 1986 Dance: Dinah's Song Choreographer: Keith Noel Dancers: Jackie Rose, Hillary Coley & Dawn Wilson
(Shaw Theatre, London)

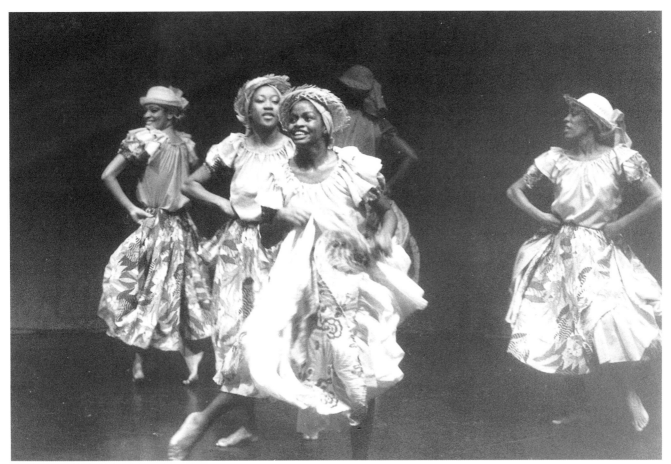

Movements Dance Company, 1986 Dance: Jamboree Choreographer: Jackie Guy Dancers: Dawn Wilson, Sharon Tai, Jackie Rose & Hillary Coley
(Spinney Hall, Northampton, England)

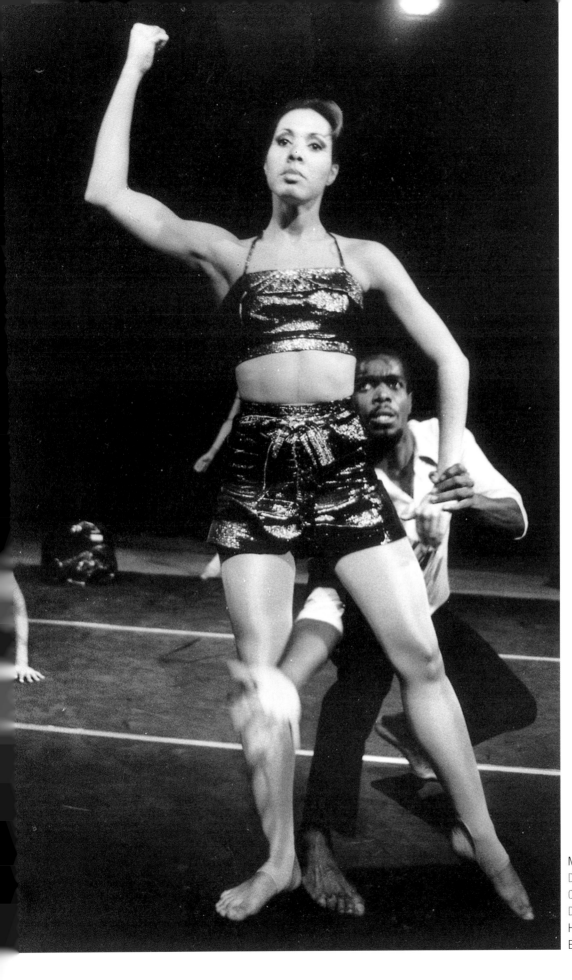

Movements Dance Company, 1986
Dance: Dinah's Song
Choreographer: Keith Noel
Dancers: Claudia Ashton & Nigel
Hinds (Leadmill Theatre, Sheffield,
England)

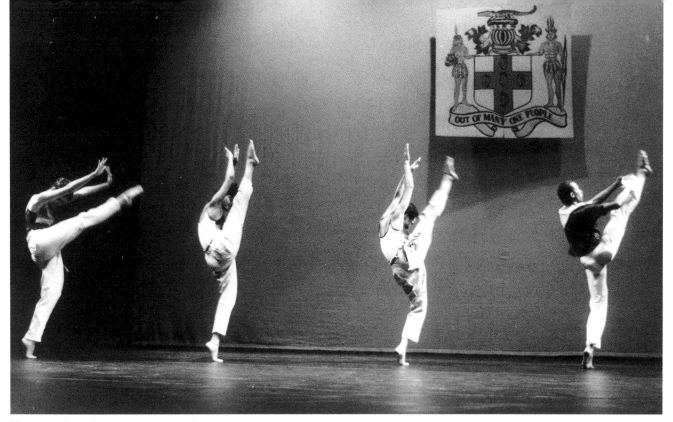

Movements Dance Company, 1986 Dance: Serenade Choreographer: Jackie Guy Dancers: Dawn Wilson, Jackie Rose, Sharon Tai & Patrick Johnson
(Shaw Theatre, London)

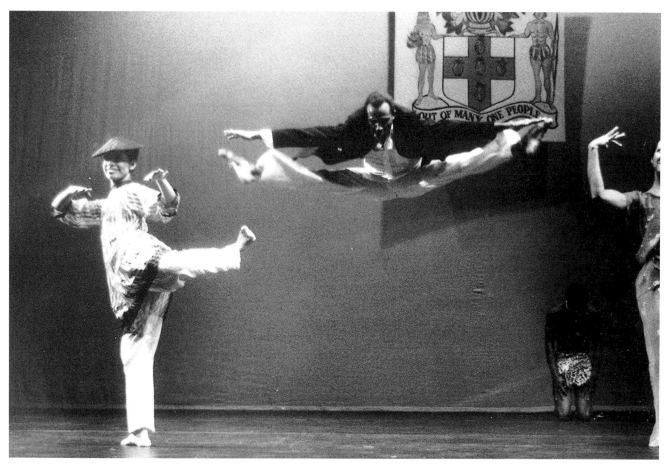

Movements Dance Company, 1986 Dance: Serenade Choreographer: Jackie Guy Dancers: Dawn Wilson, Patrick Johnson & Claudia Ashton
(Shaw Theatre, London)

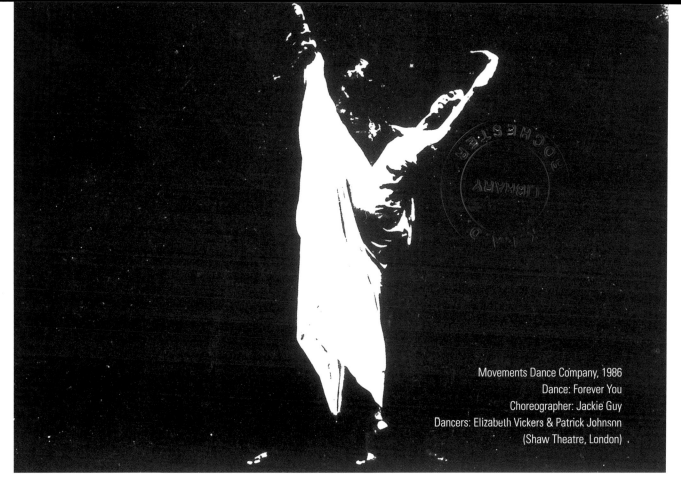

Movements Dance Company, 1986
Dance: Forever You
Choreographer: Jackie Guy
Dancers: Elizabeth Vickers & Patrick Johnson
(Shaw Theatre, London)

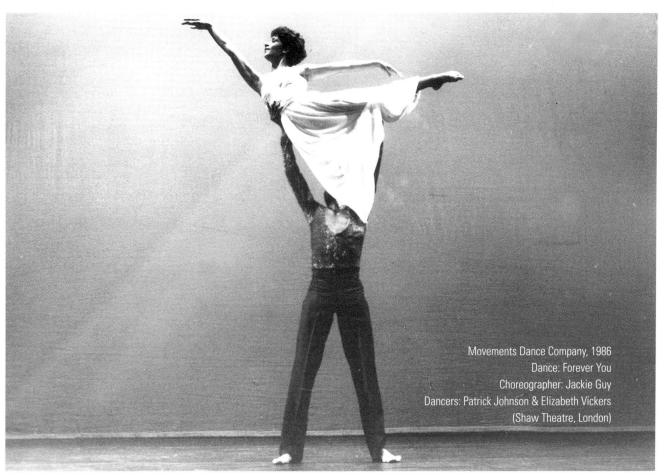

Movements Dance Company, 1986
Dance: Forever You
Choreographer: Jackie Guy
Dancers: Patrick Johnson & Elizabeth Vickers
(Shaw Theatre, London)

Movements Dance Company, 1987
Dance: Lilac Blossom
Choreographer: Monica Campbell
Dancer: Elizabeth Vickers

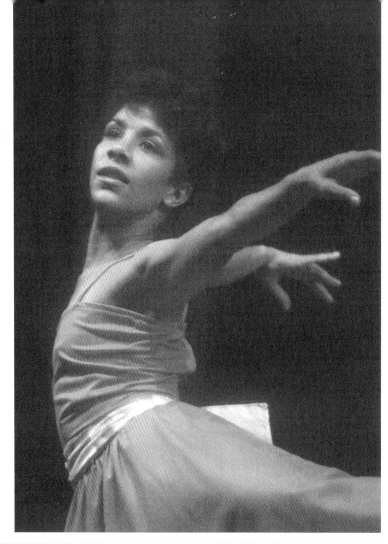

Movements Dance Company, 1987
Dance: Lilac Blossom
Choreographer: Monica Campbell
Dancer: Karin Wilson

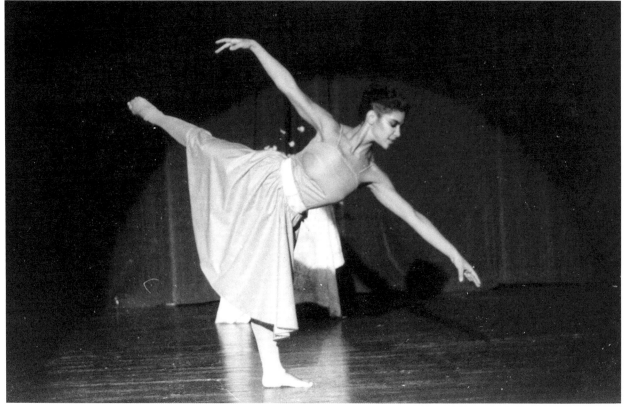

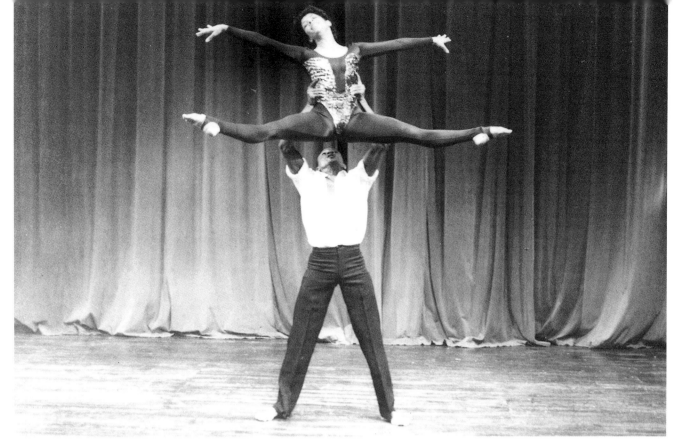

Movements Dance Company, 1987 Dance: Magic Moments Choreographer: Elizabeth Vickers Dancers: Elizabeth Vickers & Patrick Johnson

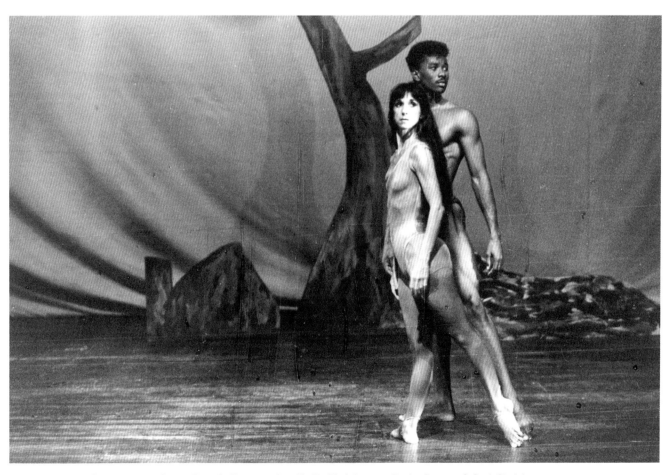

Movements Dance Company, 1987 Dance: Genesis Choreographer: Neville Black Dancers: Denise Desnoes & Garth Sinclair

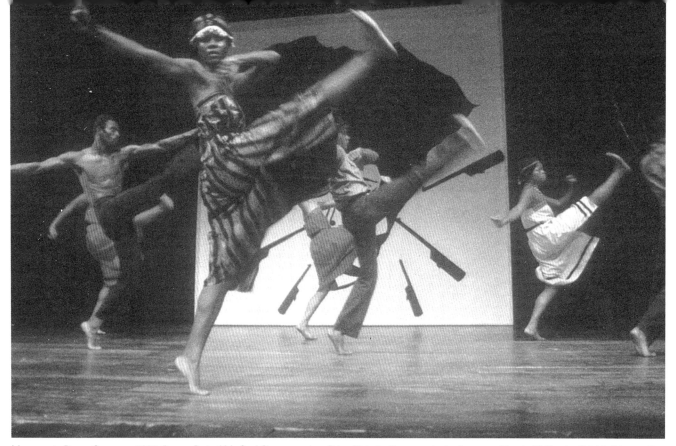

Movements Dance Company, 1987 Dance: Part of My Soul Choreographer: Patsy Ricketts Dancers: Junior Foreman, Marcia McKenzie, Patrick Johnson & Jackie Rose

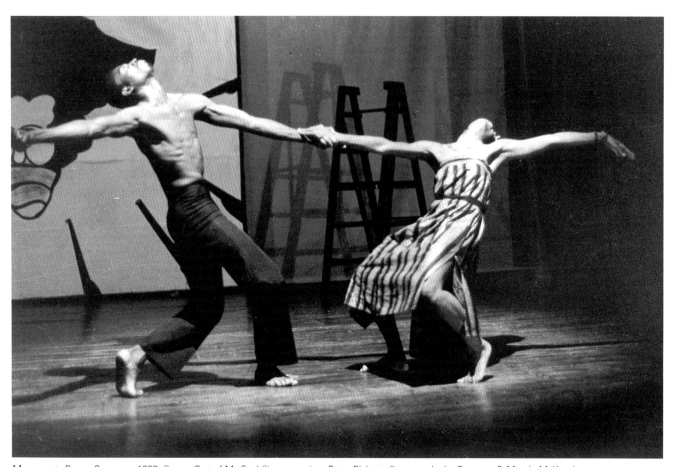

Movements Dance Company, 1987 Dance: Part of My Soul Choreographer: Patsy Ricketts Dancers: Junior Foreman & Marcia McKenzie

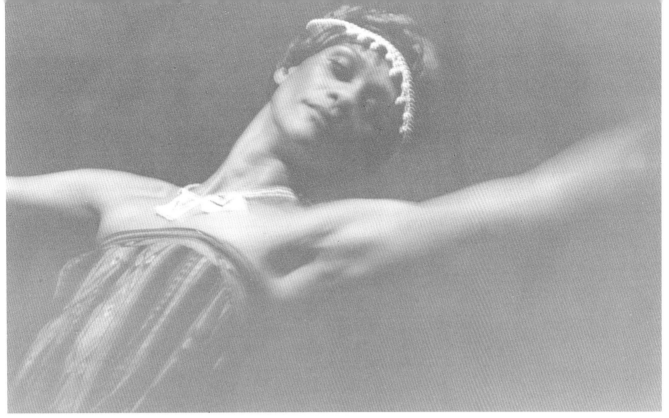

Movements Dance Company, 1988 Dance: Part of My Soul Choreographer: Patsy Ricketts Dancer: Michelle Tappin Lee

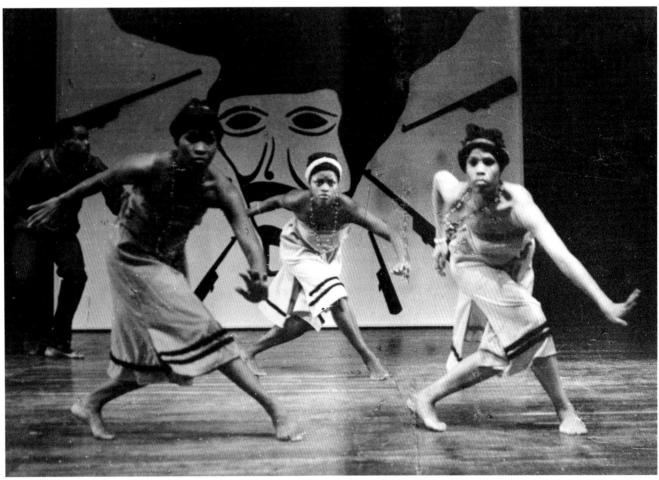

Movements Dance Company, 1988 Dance: Part of My Soul Choreographer: Patsy Ricketts Dancers: Nigel Hinds, Pat Grant, Jackie Rose &
Jennifer Harris-Bailey

Movements Dance Company, 1988
Dance: Missioner
Choreographer: Jackie Guy
Dancer: Patrick Johnson

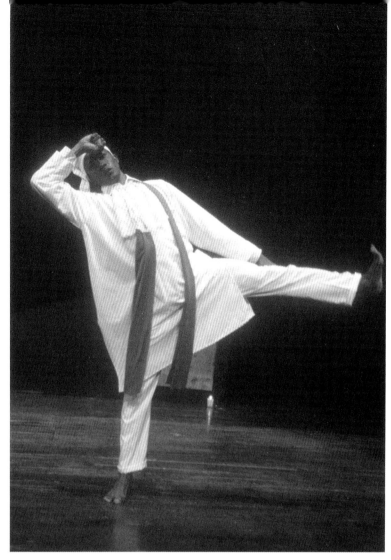

Movements Dance Company, 1988
Dance: Missioner
Choreographer: Jackie Guy
Dancers: Patrick Johnson & Company

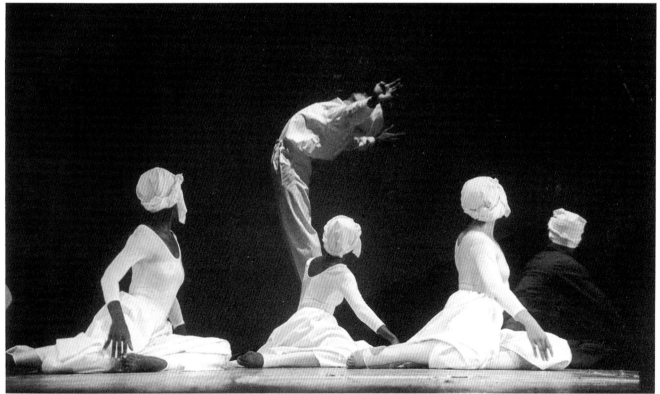

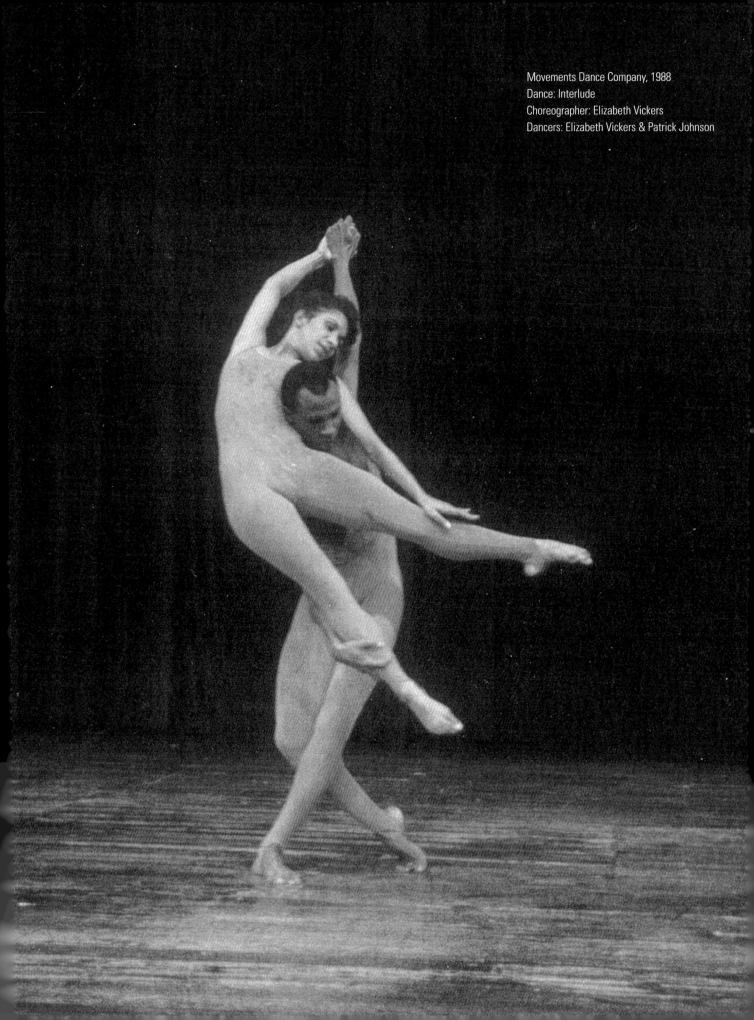

Movements Dance Company, 1988
Dance: Interlude
Choreographer: Elizabeth Vickers
Dancers: Elizabeth Vickers & Patrick Johnson

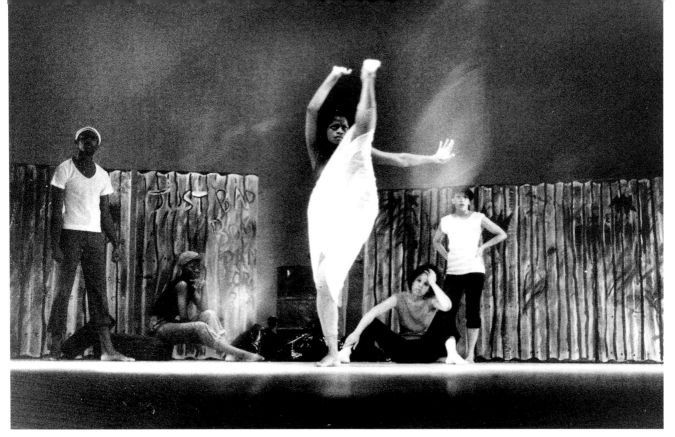

Movements Dance Company, 1989 Dance: Pressure Choreographer: Monica Campbell Dancers: Junior Foreman, Marcia McKenzie, Jackie Rose, Jennifer Harris-Bailey & Elizabeth Vickers

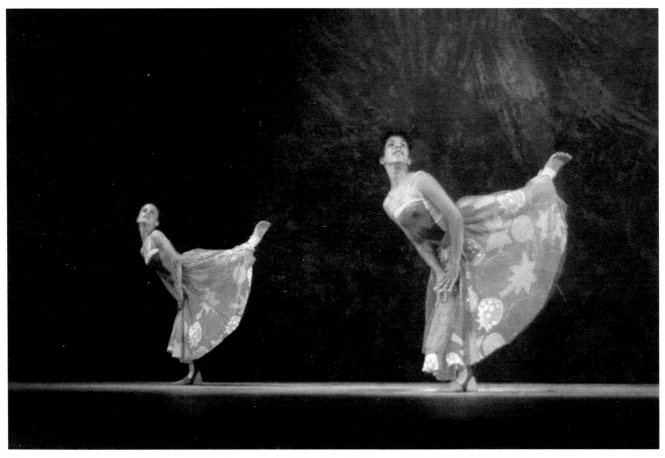

Movements Dance Company, 1989 Dance: Shades Choreographer: Monica Campbell Dancers: Keisha Steele & Elizabeth Vickers

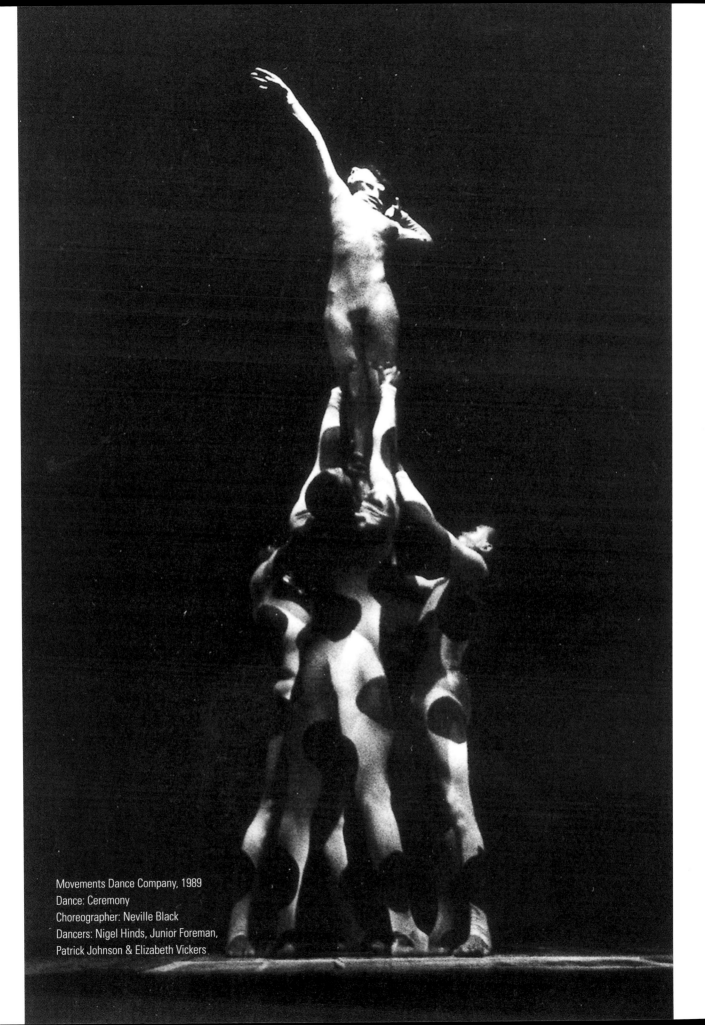

Movements Dance Company, 1989
Dance: Ceremony
Choreographer: Neville Black
Dancers: Nigel Hinds, Junior Foreman,
Patrick Johnson & Elizabeth Vickers

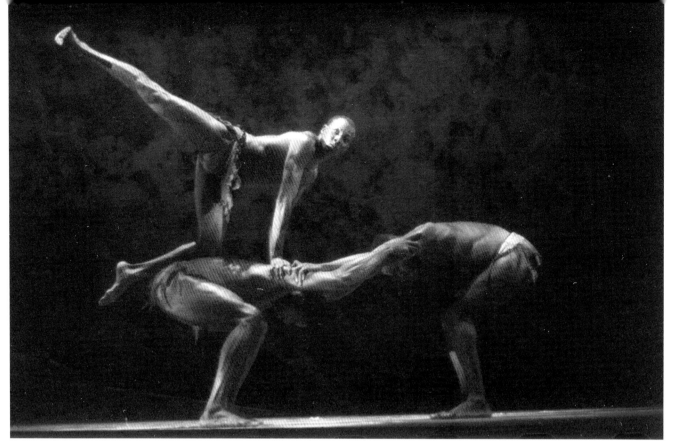

Movements Dance Company, 1989 Dance: Ceremony Choreographer: Neville Black Dancers: Patrick Johnson, Junior Foreman & Nigel Hinds

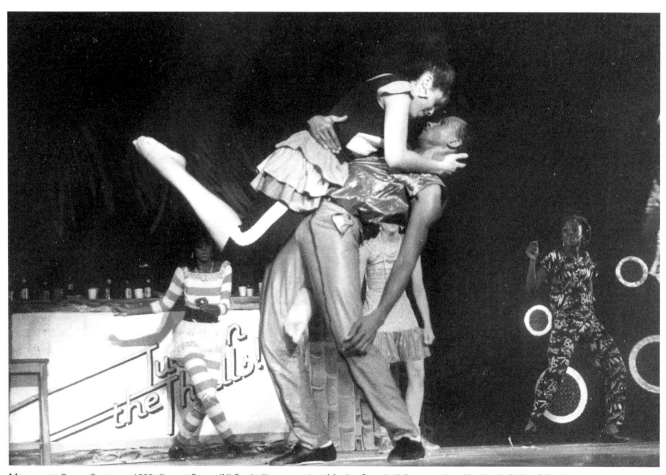

Movements Dance Company, 1989 Dance: Cease 'N' Settle Choreographer: Monica Campbell Dancers: Jennifer Harris-Bailey & Patrick Johnson

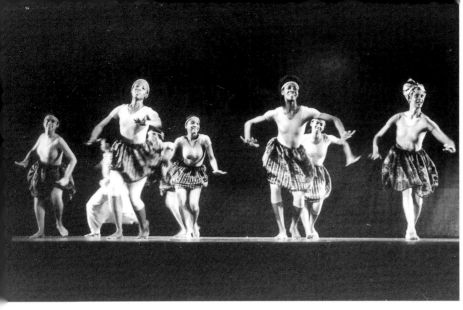

Movements Dance Company, 1991
Dance: Transitions
Choreographer: Jackie Guy
Dancers: Raquel Dunbar, Shelley Stone-Beek, Simone Thompson, Marcia McKenzie, Nikita Edwards & Michelle Tappin-Lee

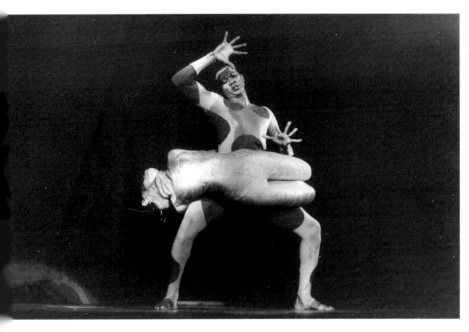

Movements Dance Company, 1991
Dance: Ceremony
Choreographer: Neville Black
Dancers: Jennifer Harris-Bailey & Patrick Johnson

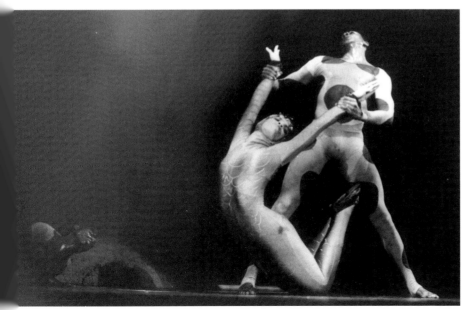

Movements Dance Company, 1991
Dance: Ceremony
Choreographer: Neville Black
Dancers: Junior Foreman, Jennifer Harris-Bailey & Patrick Johnson

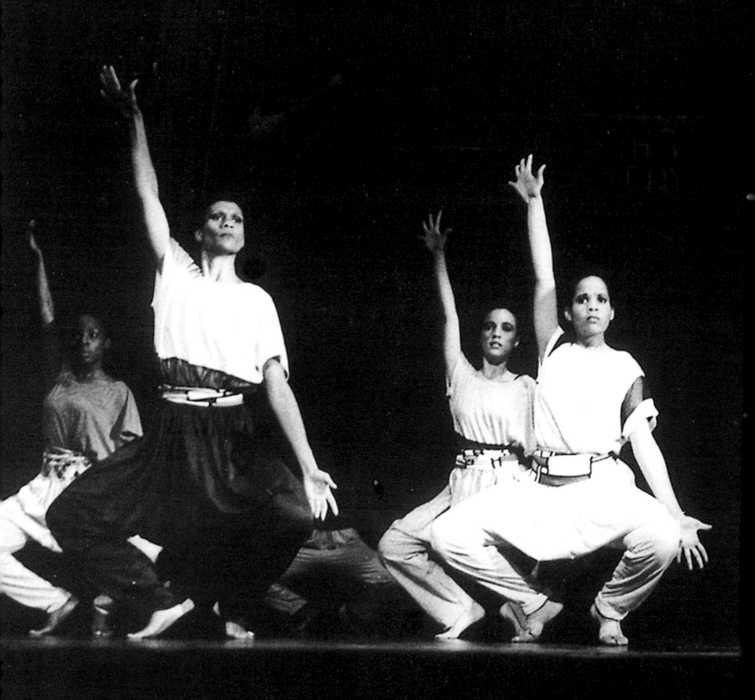

Movements Dance Company, 1991
Dance: Times and Themes
Choreographer: Monica Campbell
Dancers: Shelley Stone-Beek, Michelle Tappin-Lee, Kamina Johnson, Jennifer Harris-Bailey,
Nigel Hinds, Patrick Johnson, Wayne Campbell & Elizabeth Vickers

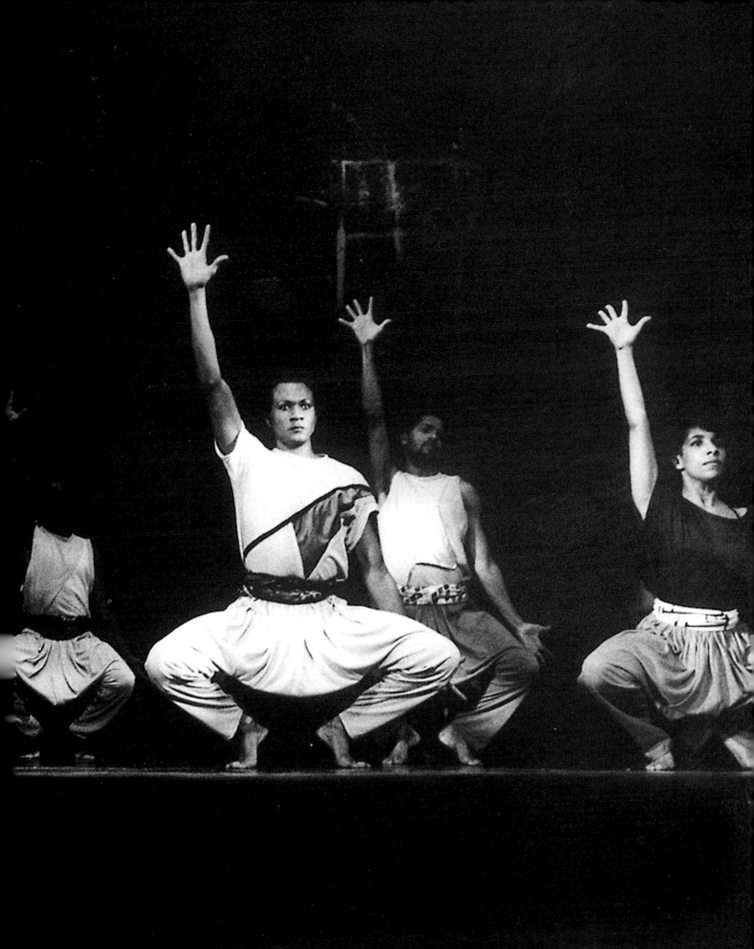

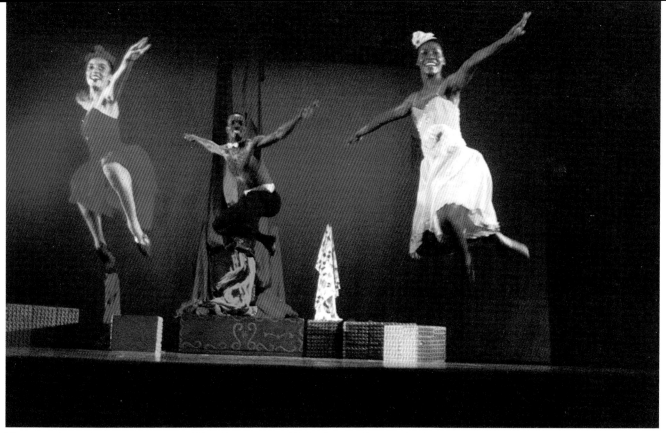

Movements Dance Company, 1991 Dance: Echings Choreographer: Monica Campbell Dancers: Kamina Johnson, Nigel Hinds & Marcia McKenzie

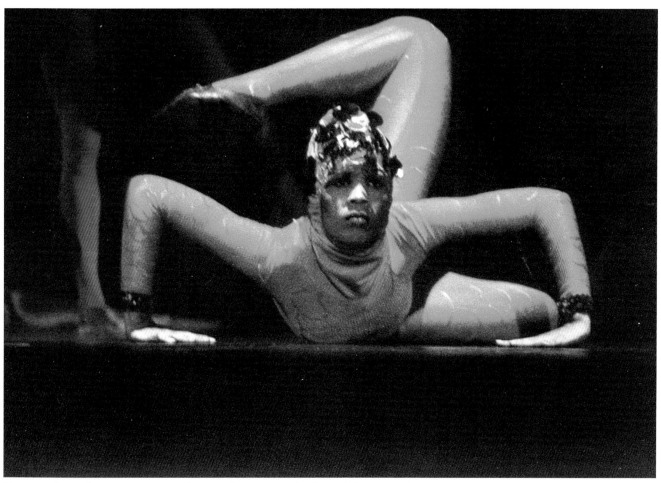

Movements Dance Company, 1991 Dance: Ceremony Choreographer: Neville Black Dancer: Jennifer Harris-Bailey

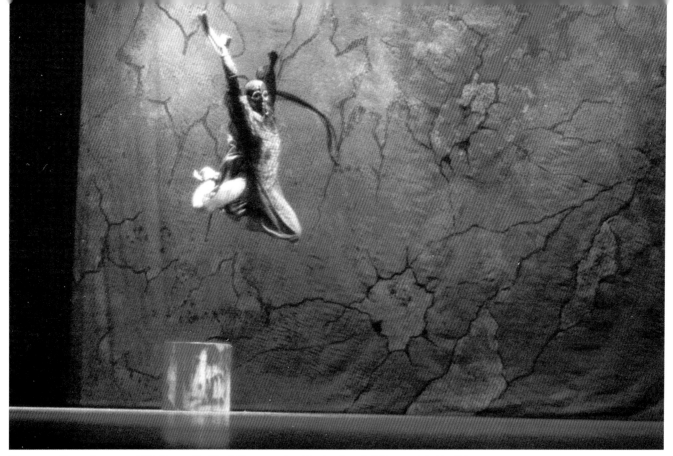

Movements Dance Company, 1993 Dance: Flashback Choreographer: Monica Campbell Dancer: Aristides Bringuez

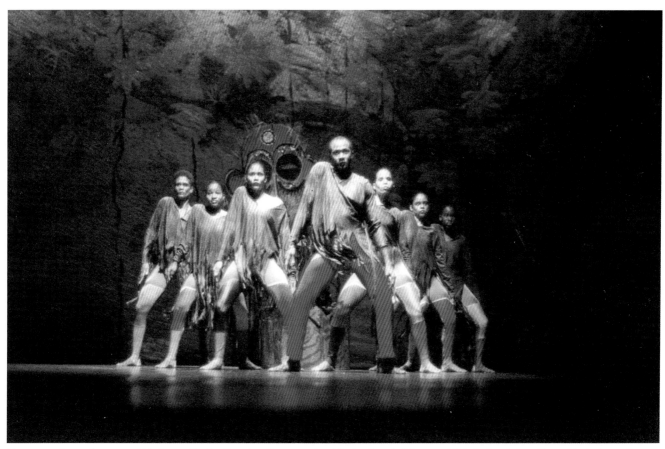

Movements Dance Company, 1993 Dance: Rhythm Branches Choreographer: Monica Campbell Dancers: Michelle Tappin-Lee, Dionne Harris, Leesa Kow, Patrick Johnson, Jennifer Harris-Bailey, Raquel Dunbar & Dionne Guthrie

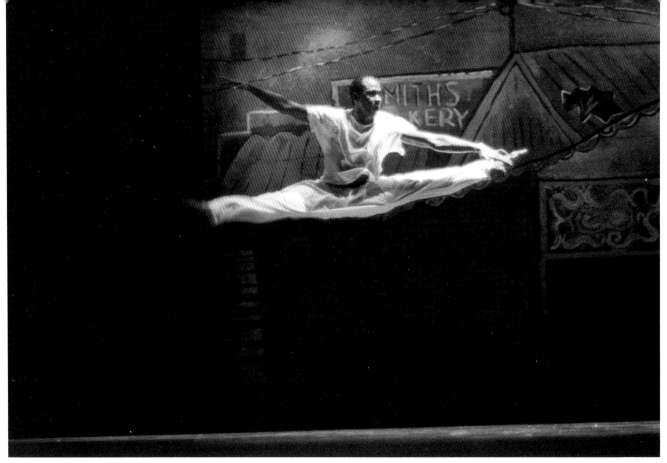

Movements Dance Company, 1993 Dance: Times and Themes Choreographer: Monica Campbell Dancer: Patrick Johnson

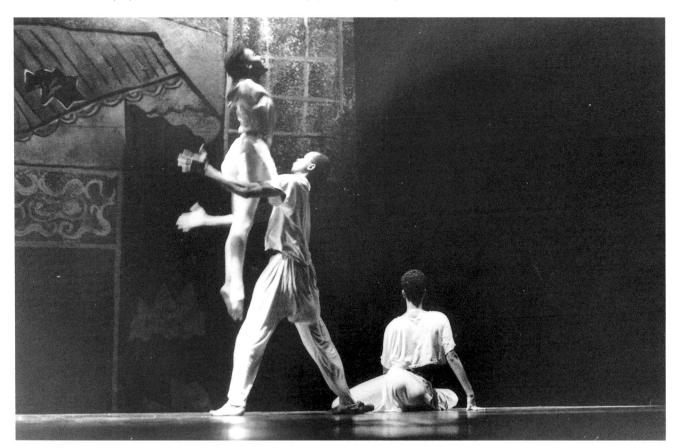

Movements Dance Company, 1993 Dance: Times and Themes Choreographer: Monica Campbell Dancers: Natalie Guthrie, Patrick Johnson & Michelle Tappin-Lee

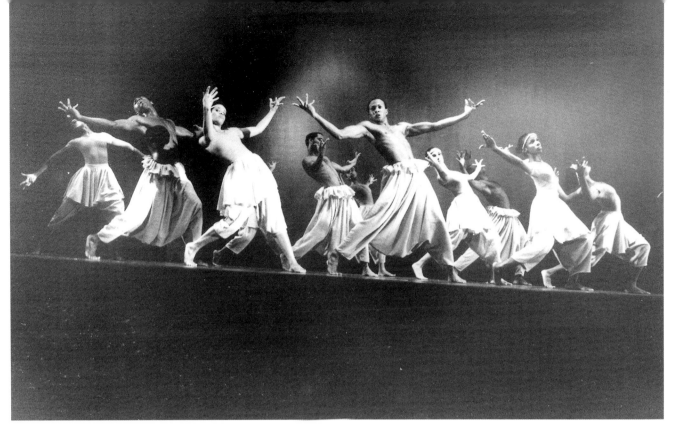

Movements Dance Company, 1993 Dance: Transitions Choreographer: Jackie Guy Dancers: The Company

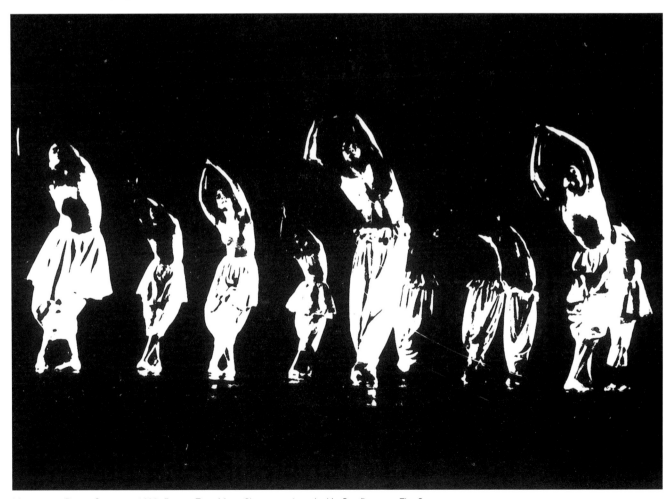

Movements Dance Company, 1993 Dance: Transitions Choreographer: Jackie Guy Dancers: The Company

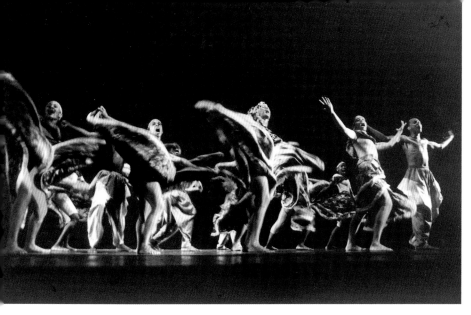

Movements Dance Company, 1993
Dance: Transitions
Choreographer: Jackie Guy
Dancers: The Company

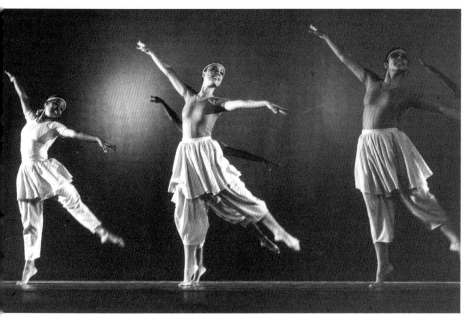

Movements Dance Company, 1994
Dance: Transitions
Choreographer: Jackie Guy
Dancers: Dionne Harris, Kamina Johnson &
Raquel Dunbar

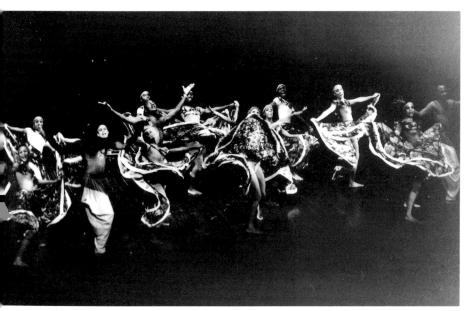

Movements Dance Company, 1994
Dance: Transitions
Choreographer: Jackie Guy
Dancers: The Company

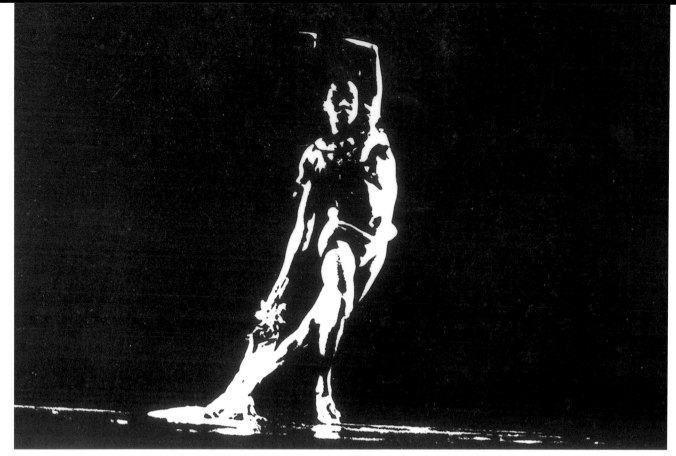

Movements Dance Company, 1993 Dance: Lotus Flower Choreographer: Vince Collins Dancer: Patrick Johnson

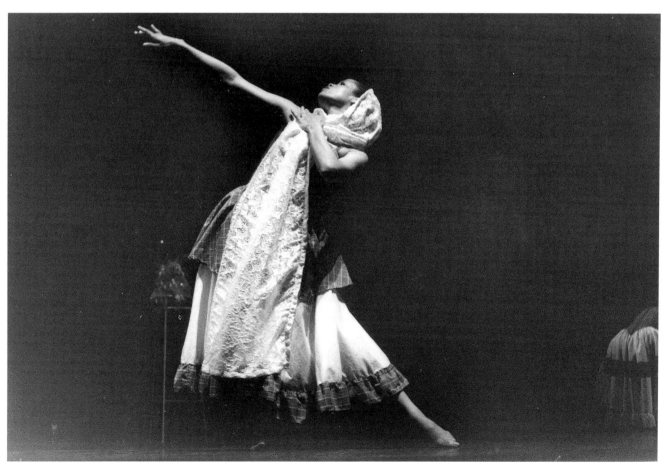

Movements Dance Company, 1993 Dance: Love Joy Choreographer: Jackie Guy Dancer: Jennifer Harris-Bailey

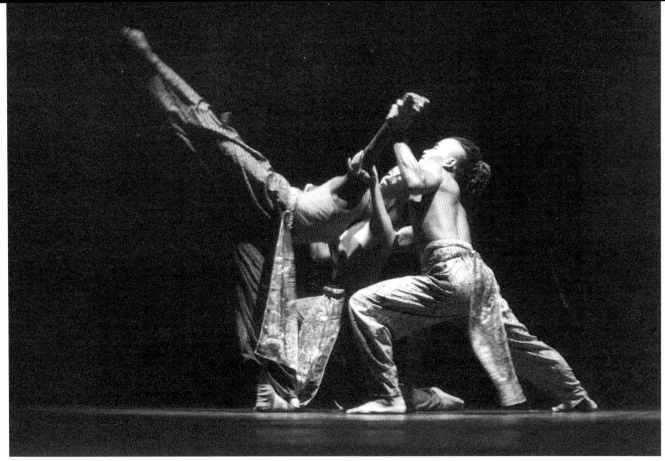

Movements Dance Company, 1993 Dance: Tik-ka Choreographer: Ray Tadio (Guest) Dancers: Natalie Guthrie, Kamina Johnson & Ray Tadio (Guest)

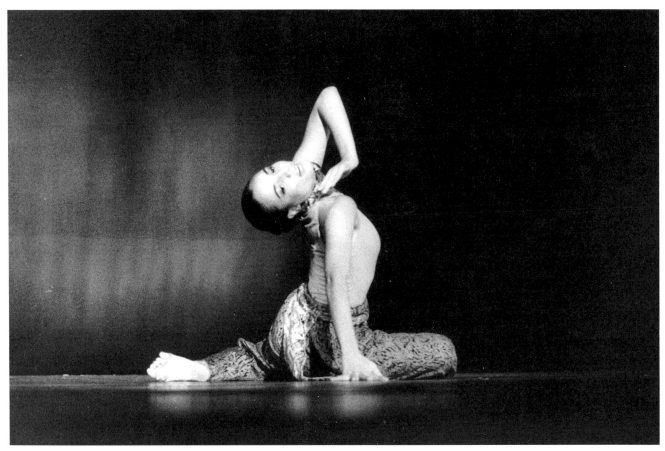

Movements Dance Company, 1993 Dance: Tik-ka Choreographer: Ray Tadio (Guest) Dancer: Kamina Johnson

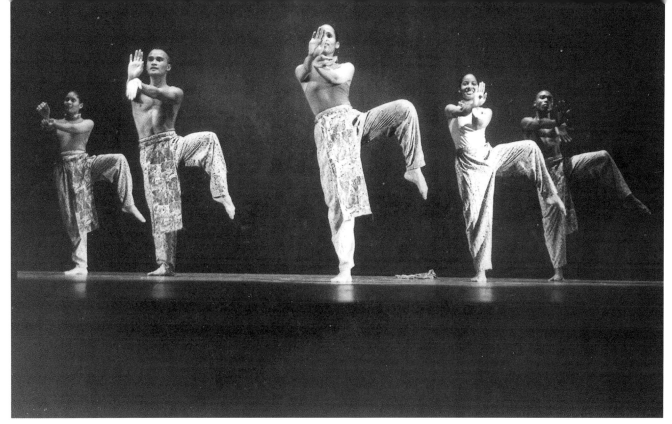

Movements Dance Company, 1993 Dance: Tik-ka Choreographer: Ray Tadio (Guest) Dancers: Leesa Kow, Ray Tadio (Guest), Jennifer Harris-Bailey, Dionne Harris & Kofi Walker

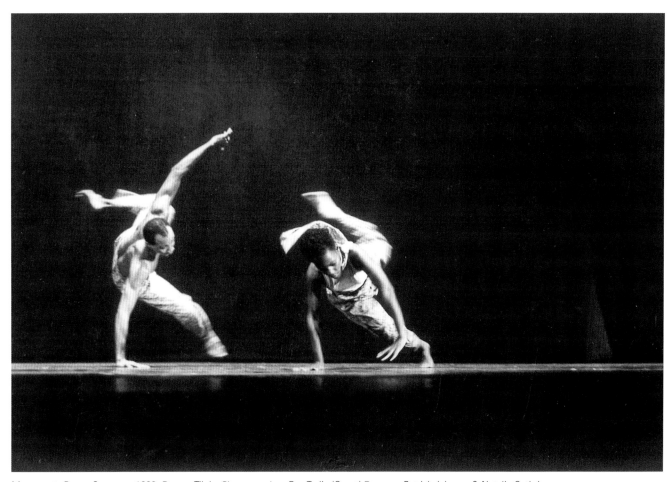

Movements Dance Company, 1993 Dance: Tik-ka Choreographer: Ray Tadio (Guest) Dancers: Patrick Johnson & Natalie Guthrie

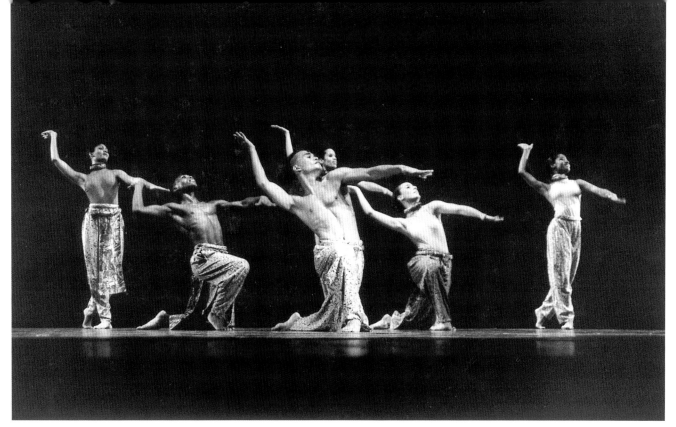

Movements Dance Company, 1993 Dance: Tik-ka Choreographer: Ray Tadio (Guest) Dancers: Leesa Kow, Kofi Walker, Ray Tadio (Guest), Jennifer Harris-Bailey, Kamina Johnson & Dionne Harris

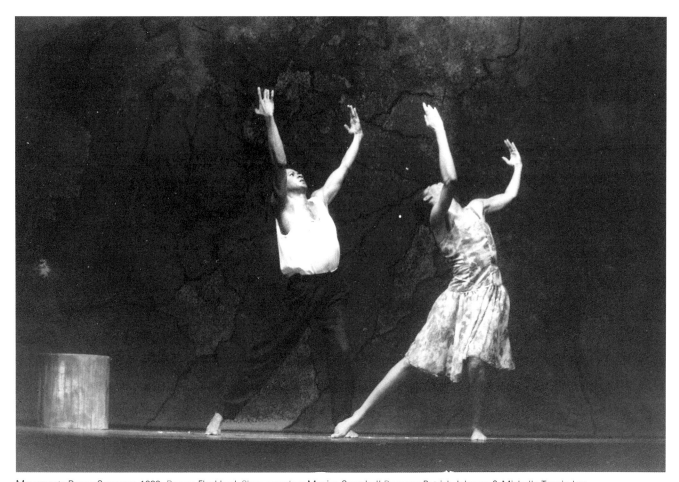

Movements Dance Company, 1993 Dance: Flashback Choreographer: Monica Campbell Dancers: Patrick Johnson & Michelle Tappin-Lee

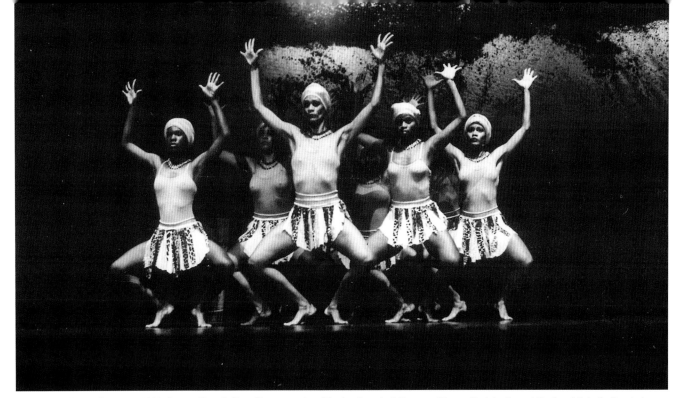

Movements Dance Company, 1994 Dance: Cosmic Beat Choreographer: Monica Campbell Dancers: Dionne Guthrie, Raquel Dunbar, Michelle Tappin-Lee, Jackie Rose & Leesa Kow

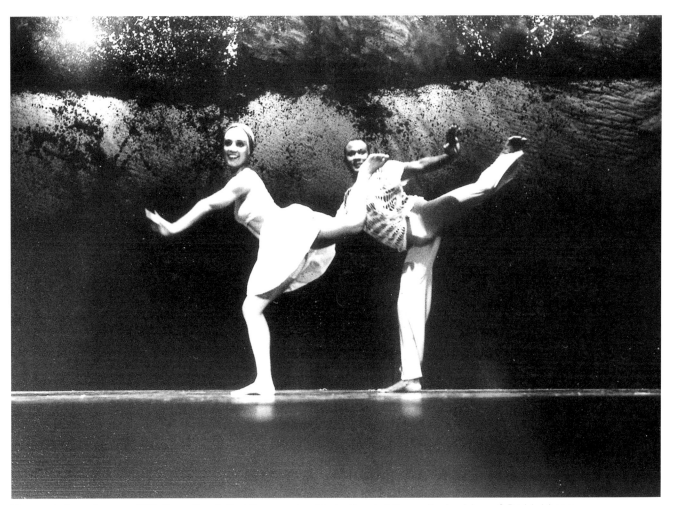

Movements Dance Company, 1994 Dance: Cosmic Beat Choreographer: Monica Campbell Dancer: Kamina Johnson & Patrick Johnson

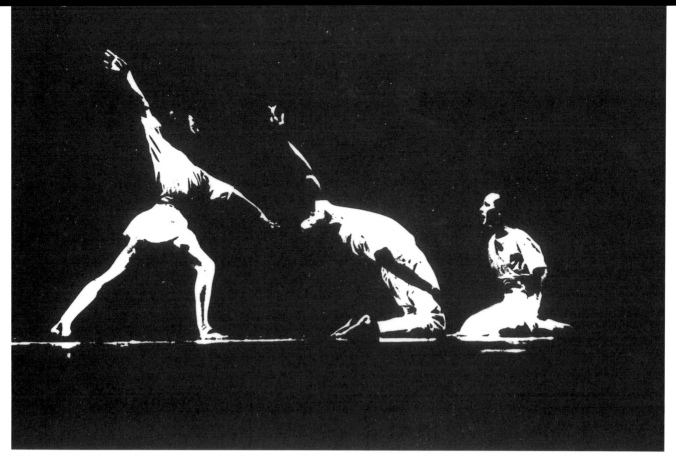

Movements Dance Company, 1994 Dance: Times and Themes Choreographer: Monica Campbell Dancers: Natalie Guthrie, Patrick Johnson & Kamina Johnson

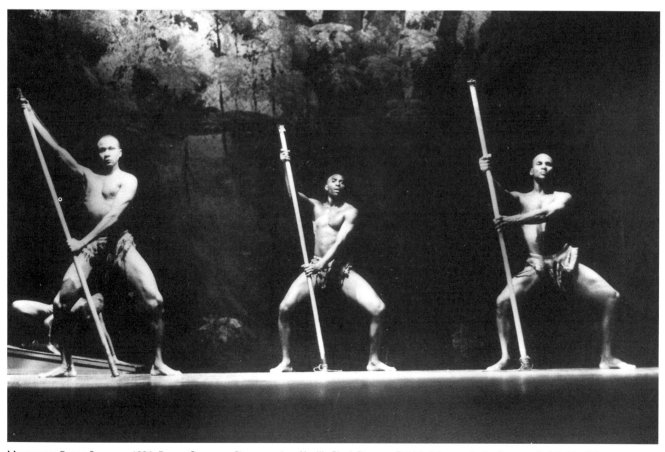

Movements Dance Company, 1994 Dance: Ceremony Choreographer: Neville Black Dancers: Patrick Johnson, Junior Foreman & Aristides Bringuez

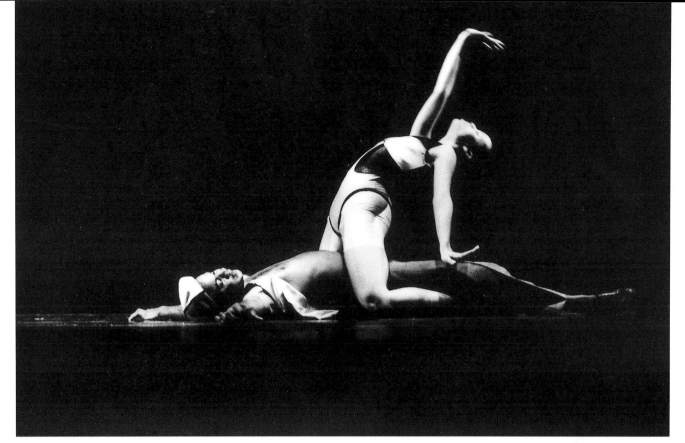

Movements Dance Company, 1994 Dance: Flashback Choreographer: Monica Campbell Dancers: Patrick Johnson & Jennifer Harris-Bailey

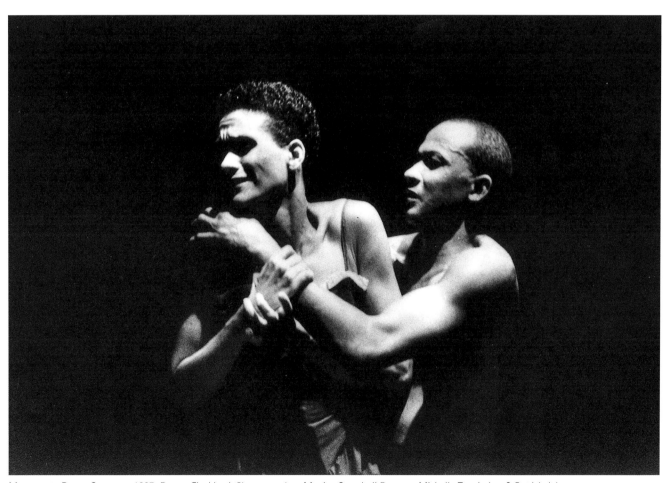

Movements Dance Company, 1995 Dance: Flashback Choreographer: Monica Campbell Dancers: Michelle Tappin-Lee & Patrick Johnson

…and in great halls

of houses great

delicately moved

the owner and his mates

to the faint music they made

and the bonded heard

and kept alive the tune

soon the music was what they played

secretly they danced too

for the memory was deep and strong

enticing those who dance in the halls

till some memories dimmed paled

but the compelling dance

continued still

urging willing

till it was freedom time…

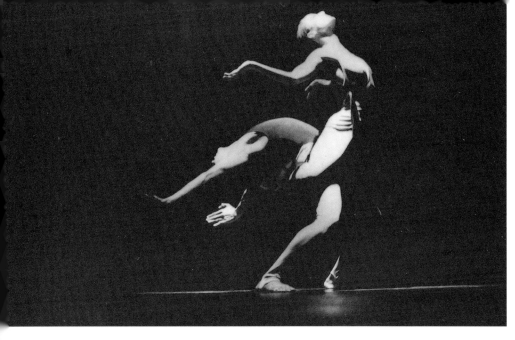

Movements Dance Company, 1995
Dance: Oshumare
Choreographer: Monica Campbell
Dancers: Patrick Johnson & Kamina Johnson

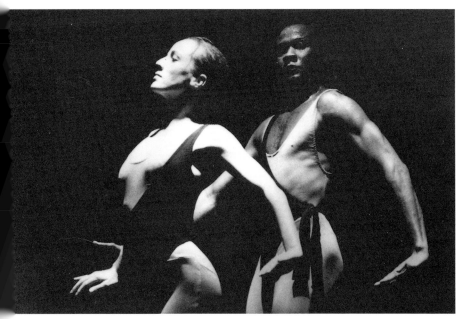

Movements Dance Company, 1995
Dance: Oshumare
Choreographer: Monica Campbell
Dancers: Kamina Johnson & Patrick Johnson

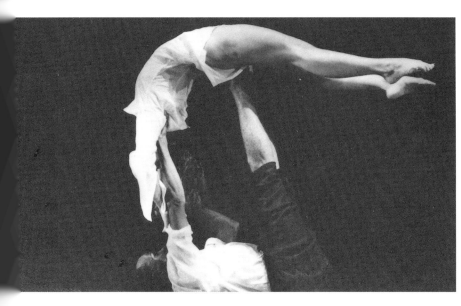

Movements Dance Company, 1995
Dance: Autumn Breeze
Choreographer: Jamel Gaines
Dancers: Patrick Johnson & Dionne Harris

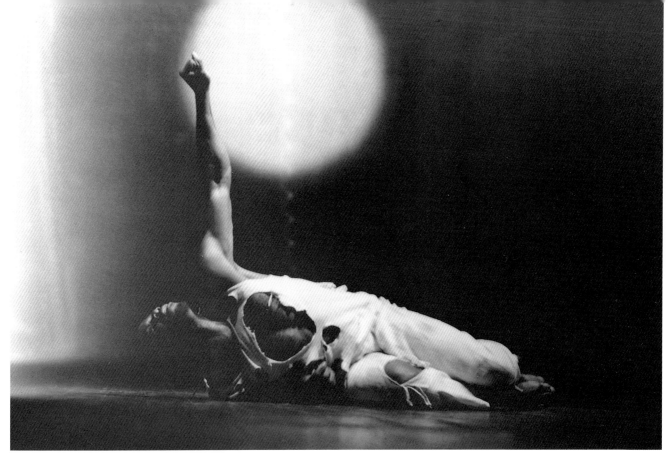

Movements Dance Company, 1995 Dance: Pressure Choreographer: Monica Campbell Dancer: Nigel Hinds

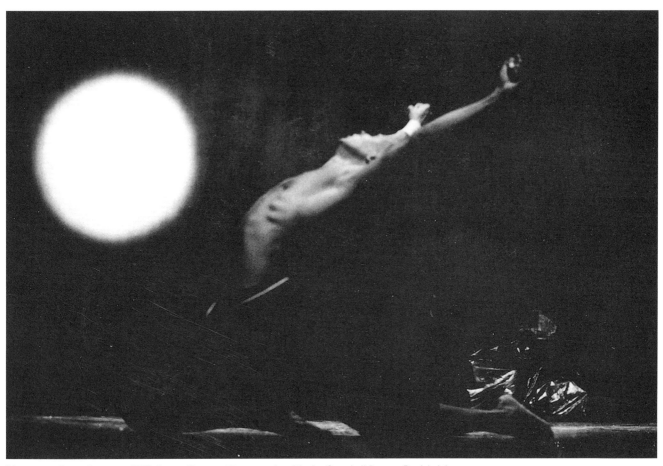

Movements Dance Company, 1995 Dance: Pressure Choreographer: Monica Campbell Dancer: Patrick Johnson

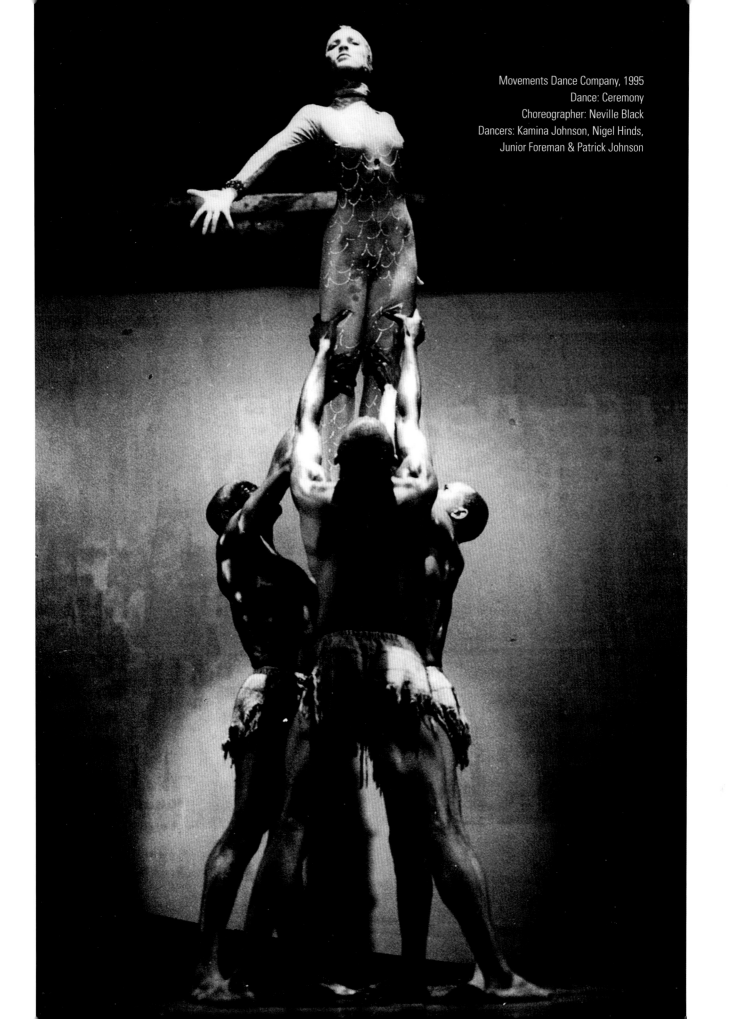

Movements Dance Company, 1995
Dance: Ceremony
Choreographer: Neville Black
Dancers: Kamina Johnson, Nigel Hinds,
Junior Foreman & Patrick Johnson

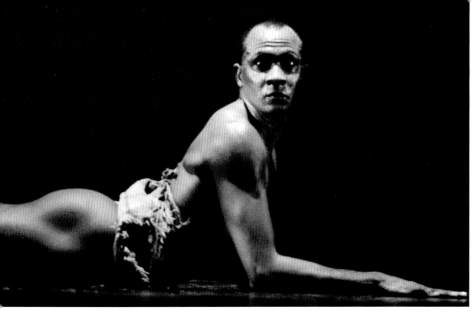

Movements Dance Company, 1995
Dance: Ceremony
Choreographer: Neville Black
Dancer: Patrick Johnson

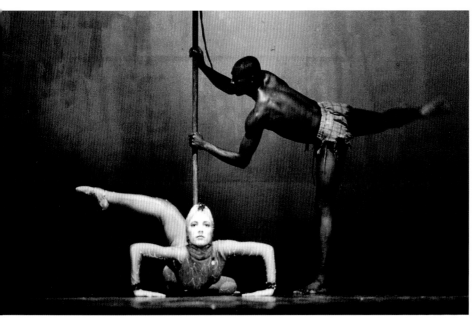

Movements Dance Company, 1995
Dance: Ceremony
Choreographer: Neville Black
Dancers: Kamina Johnson & Junior Foreman

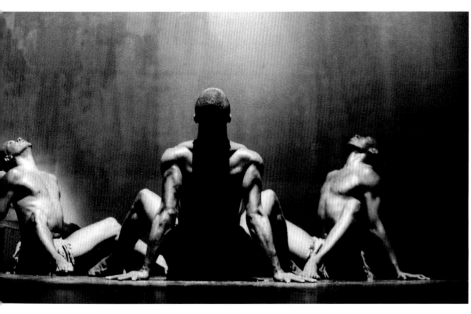

Movements Dance Company, 1995
Dance: Ceremony
Choreographer: Neville Black
Dancers: Patrick Johnson, Nigel Hinds & Junior Foreman

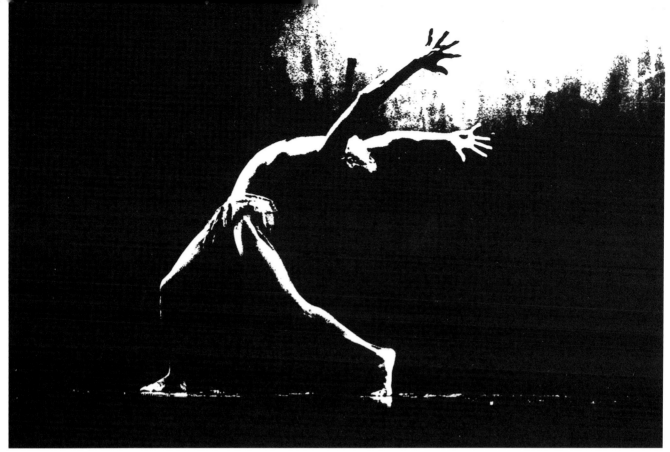

Movements Dance Company, 1995 Dance: Ceremony Choreographer: Neville Black Dancer: Patrick Johnson

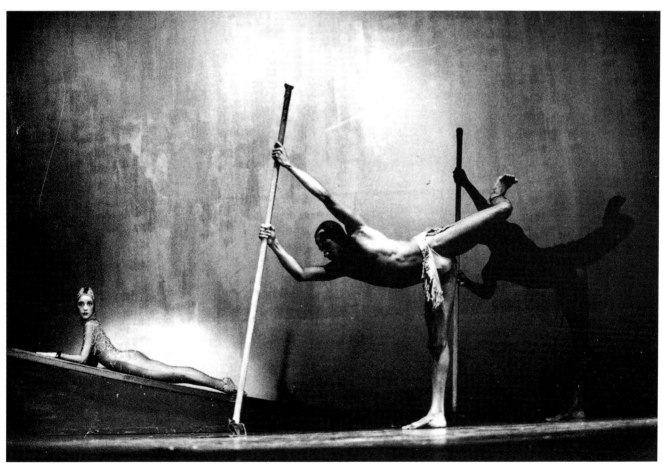

Movements Dance Company, 1995 Dance: Ceremony Choreographer: Neville Black Dancers: Kamina Johnson, Patrick Johnson & Junior Foreman

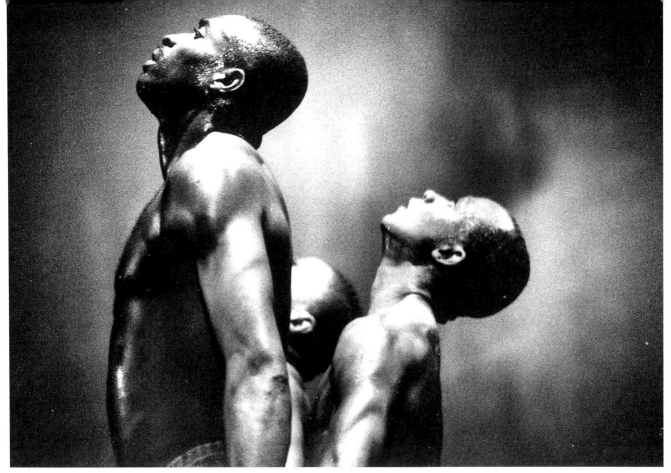

Movements Dance Company, 1995 Dance: Ceremony Choreographer: Neville Black Dancers: Junior Foreman, Nigel Hinds (partly hidden), Patrick Johnson

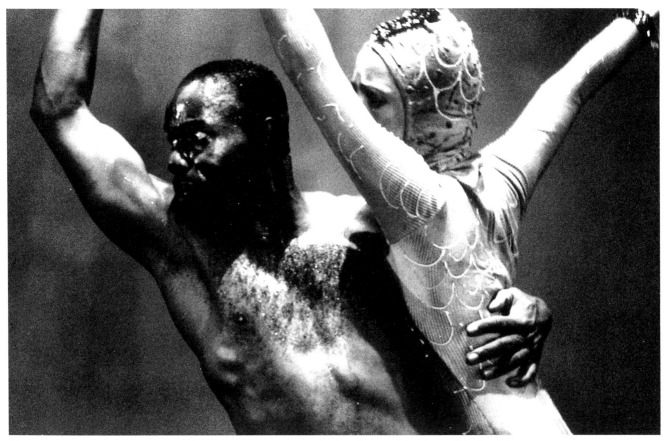

Movements Dance Company, 1995 Dance: Ceremony Choreographer: Neville Black Dancers: Nigel Hinds & Kamina Johnson

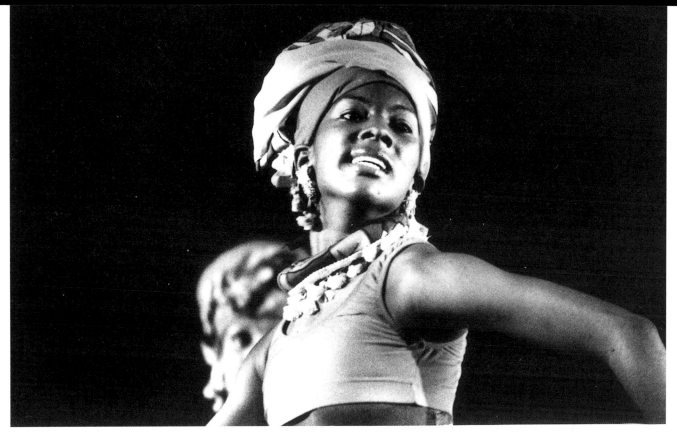

Movements Dance Company, 1995 Dance: Oshumare Choreographer: Monica Campbell Dancer: Dionne Guthrie

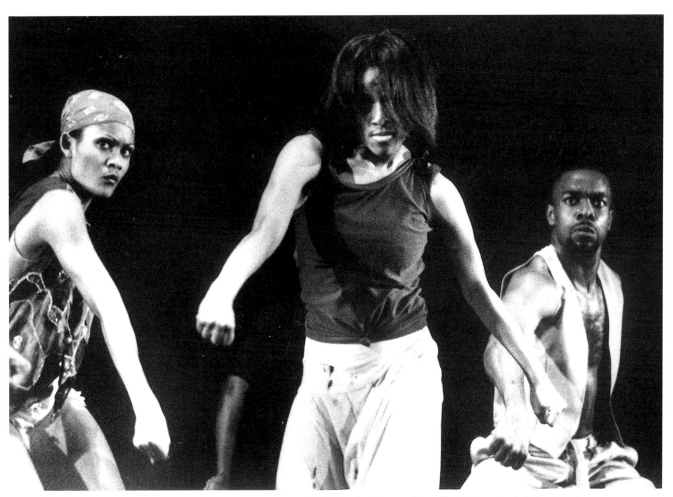

Movements Dance Company, 1995 Dance: Pressure Choreographer: Monica Campbell Dancers: Leesa Kow, Dionne Harris & Nigel Hinds

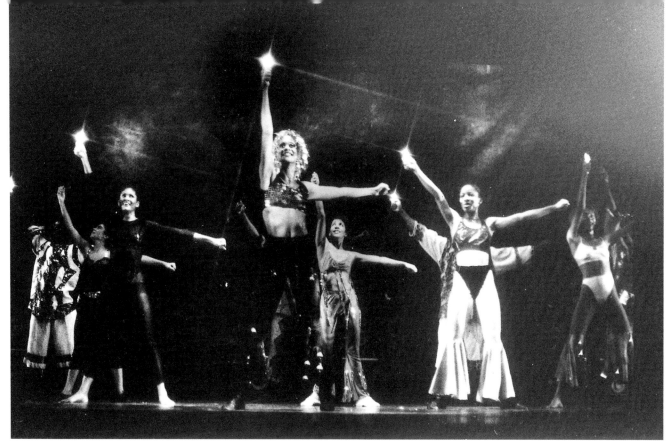

Movements Dance Company, 1995 Dance: Cosmic Beat Choreographer: Monica Campbell Dancers: The Company

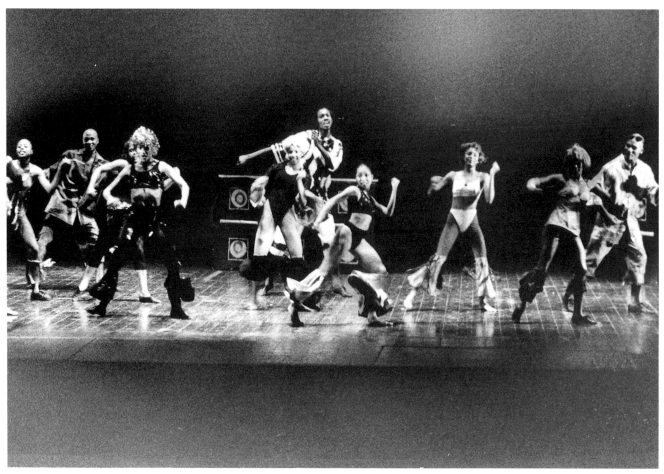

Movements Dance Company, 1996 Dance: Cosmic Beat Choreographer: Monica Campbell Dancers: The Company

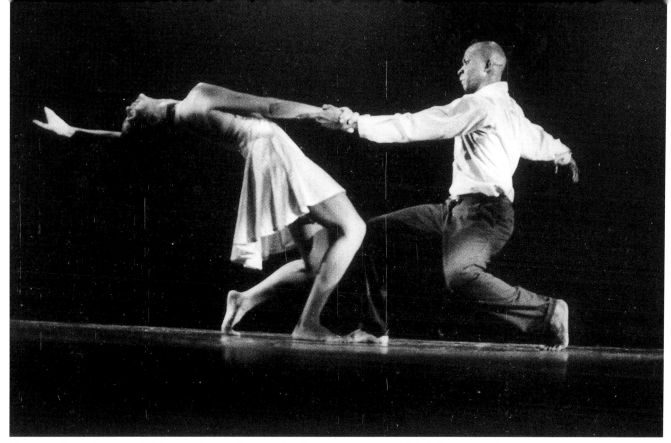

Movements Dance Company, 1996 Dance: Take Two Choreographer: Neville Black Dancers: Michelle Tappin-Lee & Patrick Johnson

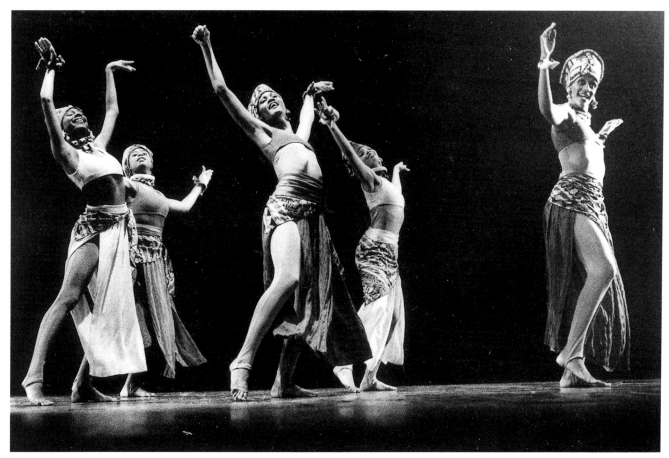

Movements Dance Company, 1996 Dance: Oshumare Choreographer: Monica Campbell Dancers: Kimberly Barrett, Michelle Morrison, Leesa Kow, Denise Harris & Michelle Tappin-Lee

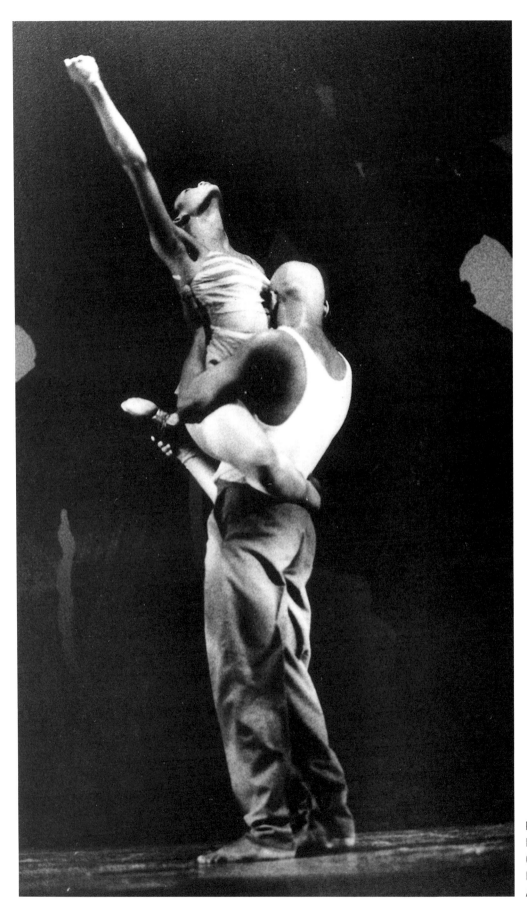

Movements Dance Company, 1996
Dance: Untold Stories
Choreographer: Monica Campbell
Dancers: Leesa Kow &
Aristides Bringuez

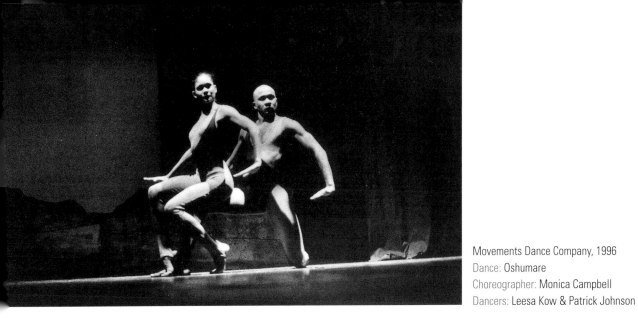

Movements Dance Company, 1996
Dance: Oshumare
Choreographer: Monica Campbell
Dancers: Leesa Kow & Patrick Johnson

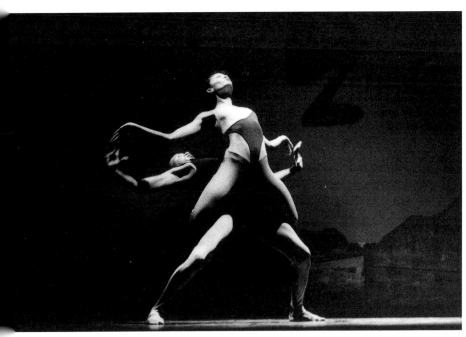

Movements Dance Company, 1996
Dance: Oshumare
Choreographer: Monica Campbell
Dancers: Patrick Johnson & Leesa Kow

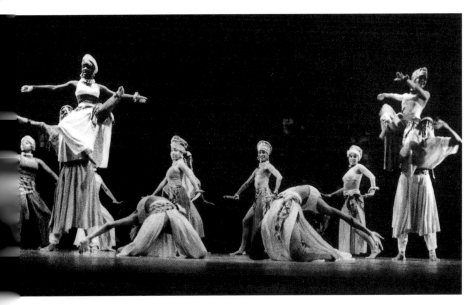

Movements Dance Company, 1996
Dance: Oshumare
Choreographer: Monica Campbell
Dancers: The Company

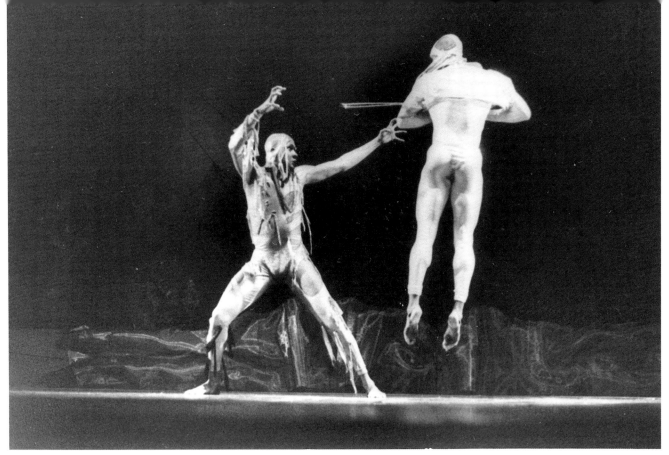

Movements Dance Company, 1998 Dance: The Rush Choreographer: Monica Campbell Dancers: Patrick Johnson & Safwan

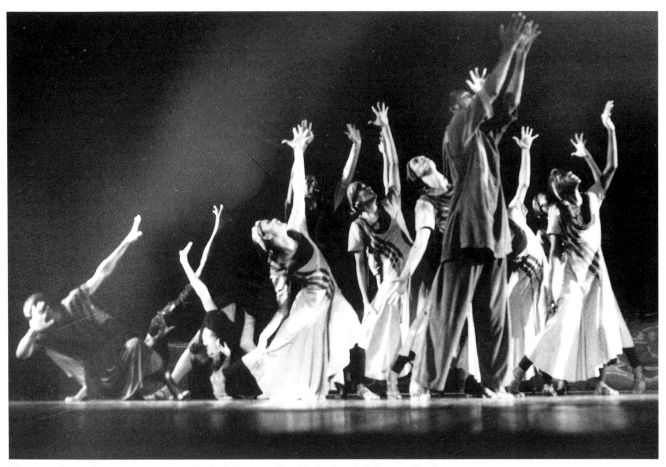

Movements Dance Company, 1998 Dance: The Rush Choreographer: Monica Campbell Dancers: The Company

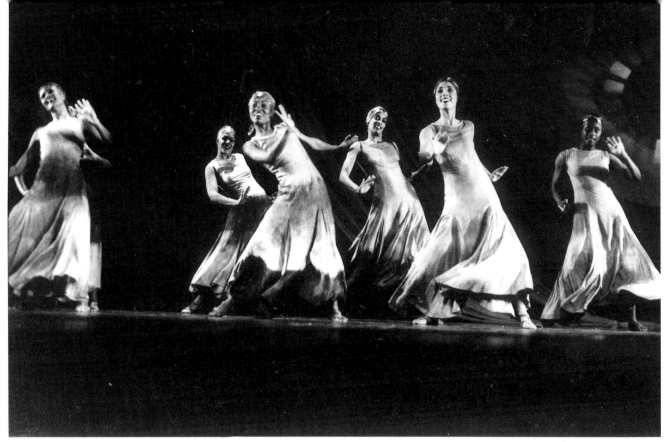

Movements Dance Company, 1998 Dance: Horizon Choreographer: Monica Campbell Dancers: The Company

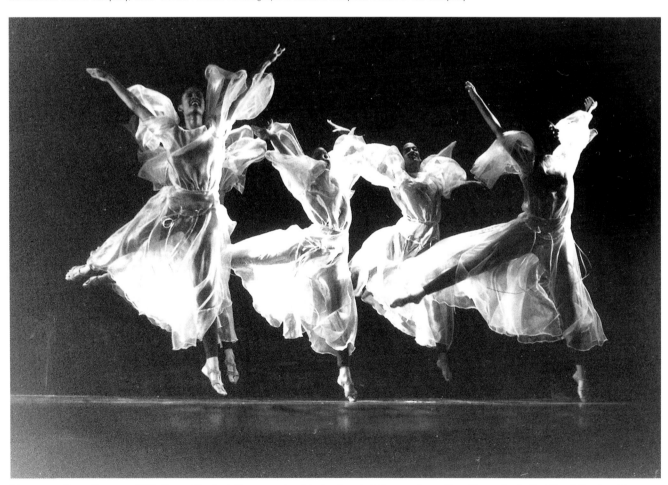

Movements Dance Company, 1998 Dance: The Rush Choreographer: Monica Campbell Dancers: Leesa Kow, Dionne Harris, Cari Diaz & Kamina Johnson

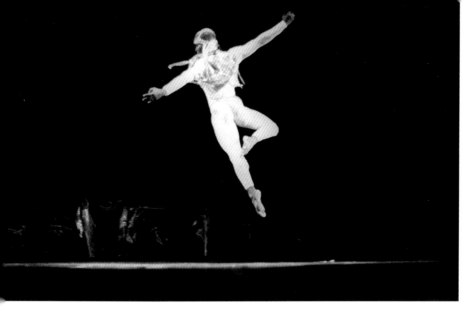

Movements Dance Company, 1998
Dance: The Rush
Choreographer: Monica Campbell
Dancer: Safwan

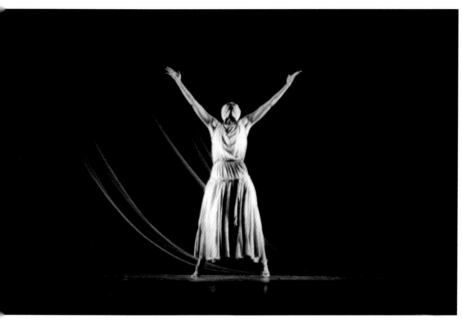

Movements Dance Company, 1998
Dance: Horizon
Choreographer: Monica Campbell
Dancer: Michelle Tappin-Lee

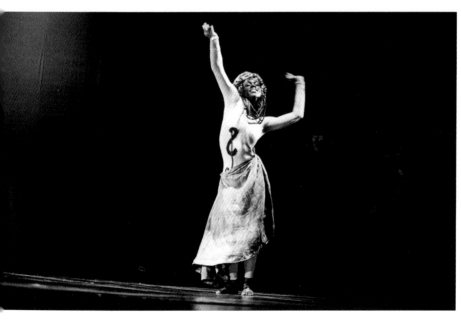

Movements Dance Company, 2002
Dance: The Mood, The Muse, The Music
Choreographer: Michael Holgate
Dancer: Dionne Guthrie

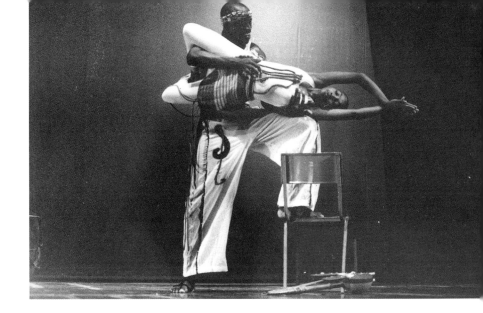

Movements Dance Company, 2002
Dance: The Mood, The Muse, The Music
Choreographer: Michael Holgate
Dancers: Clara Kahwa & Kevin Gordon

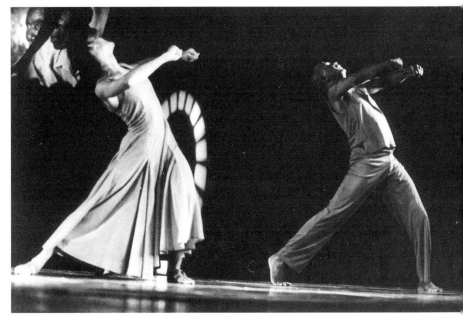

Movements Dance Company, 2002
Dance: Chosen
Choreographer: Monica Campbell
Dancers: Leesa Kow & Patrick Johnson

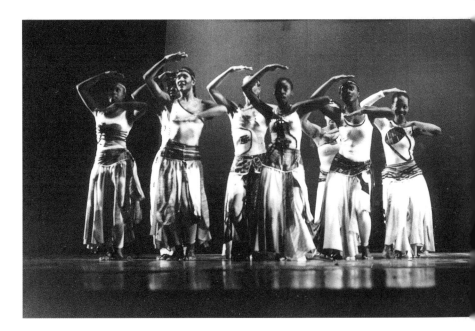

Movements Dance Company, 2002
Dance: The Mood, The Muse, The Music
Choreographer: Michael Holgate
Dancers: The Company

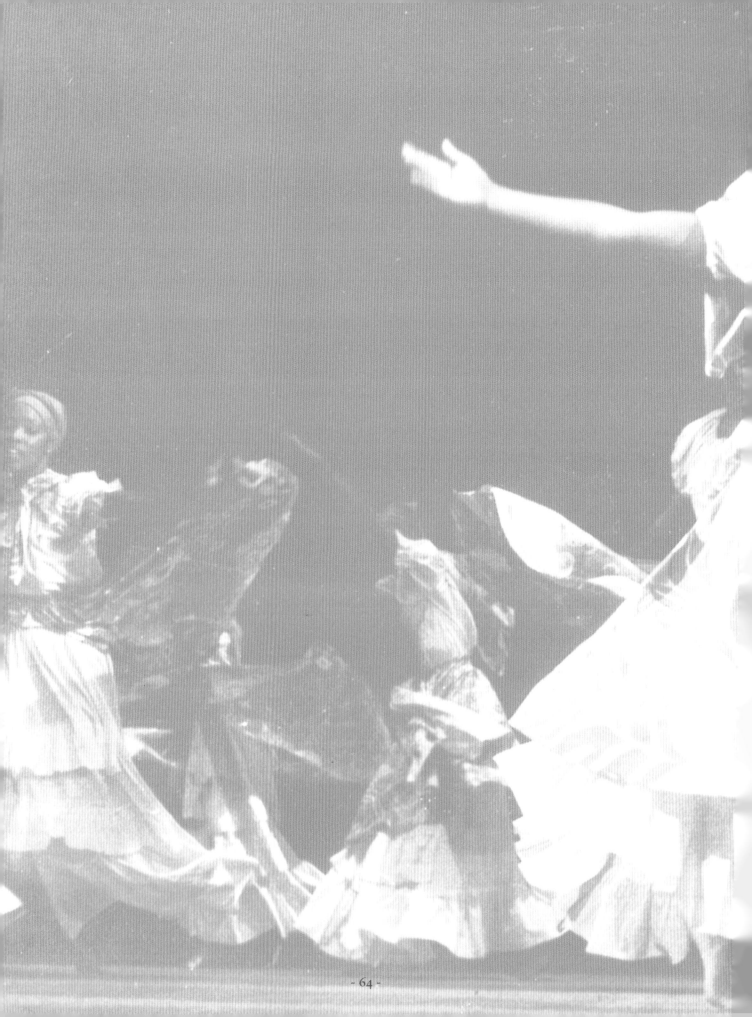

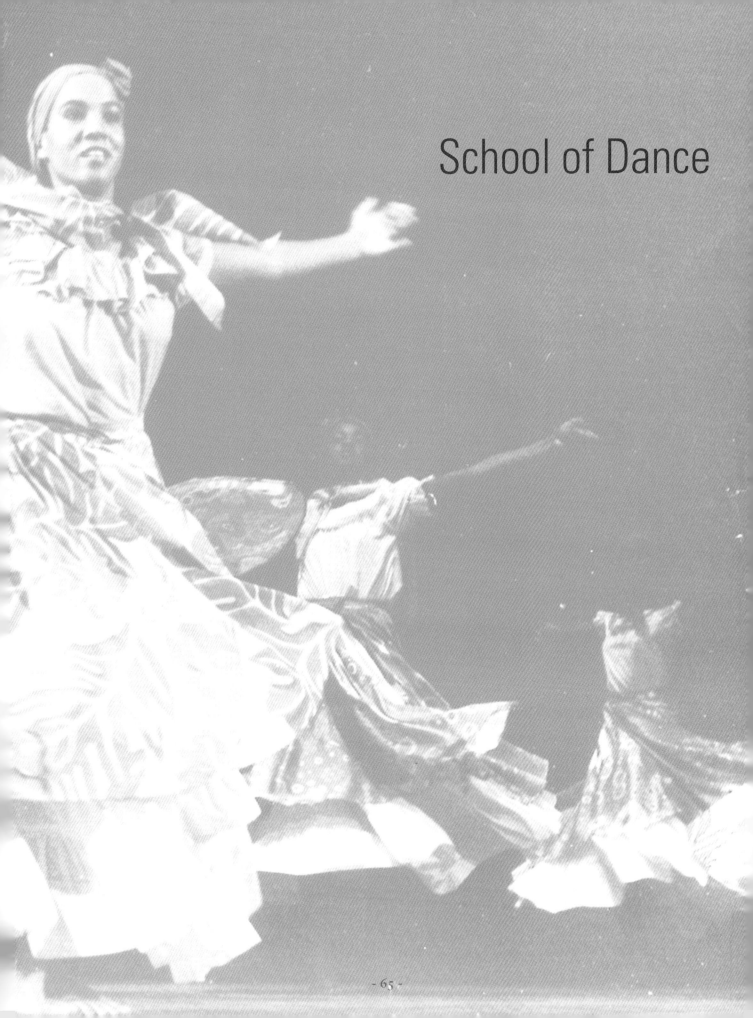

School of Dance

School of Dance

In the late 1960s, Sheila Barnett and Barbara Requa started the Contemporary Dance Centre (CDC). They were both trained as physical education teachers and were also founding members and principal dancers of The National Dance Theatre Company of Jamaica. The Contemporary Dance Centre offered two areas of training: education courses for physical education teachers interested in dance, and a programme for children aged 4 to 18 years. Shelia Barnett was the co-ordinator for the adult section and Barbara Requa co-ordinated the junior section. In 1976, Sheila Barnett, Barbara Requa and Bert Rose formed the Jamaica School of Dance, in collaboration with The National Dance Theatre Company. This school was to not only offer classes for the company dancers, but also train choreographers, instructors and dance educators for the wider society.

At first classes were conducted in a shed built by The National Dance Theatre Company on property donated by the Jamaican government. Sheila Barnett, Barbara Requa and Bert Rose were assisted by teachers from The National Dance Theatre Company, and offered classes in educational dance for teachers, studio methods and the Laban methodology for teaching children. There was a strong focus in research and training in African and Afro-Caribbean dance forms.

In 1975, the Cultural Training Centre was established by the government of Jamaica as a national centre for the arts. The School of Dance was incorporated into this centre under the direction of Sheila Barnett; Barbara Requa was the administrator and head of the junior division, and Bert Rose was the senior instructor and head of the performance department.

Over the past three decades the School of Dance has grown, establishing new programmes and associations, while providing high quality training in all aspects of teacher education and performance skills for young Jamaicans and students from the Caribbean islands, Guyana and Suriname. Graduates have gone on to do further studies and many have returned to work as lecturers. The School of Dance is currently developing a Bachelors Degree (BFA) in collaboration with the School of Music and Drama.

Barbara Requa, Co-founder

…Now the drums of Africa

play the melodies of Europe

to their beat…

bodies born of such sweet harmony

leap and bend and turn

carve the space around

rendering it their own

weaving tapestry rich

unique rainbowed beautiful

as so they mark the sound

dancing praise songs

of ancestral spirits

to their honour and delight…

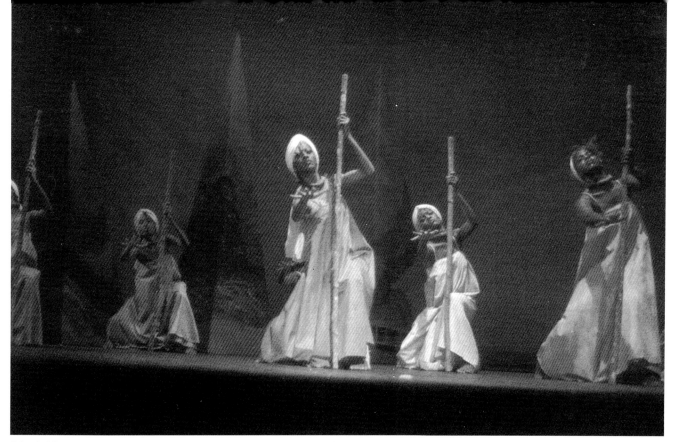

School of Dance, 1985 Dance: Voices Choreographer: Tony Wilson Dancers: The Workshop

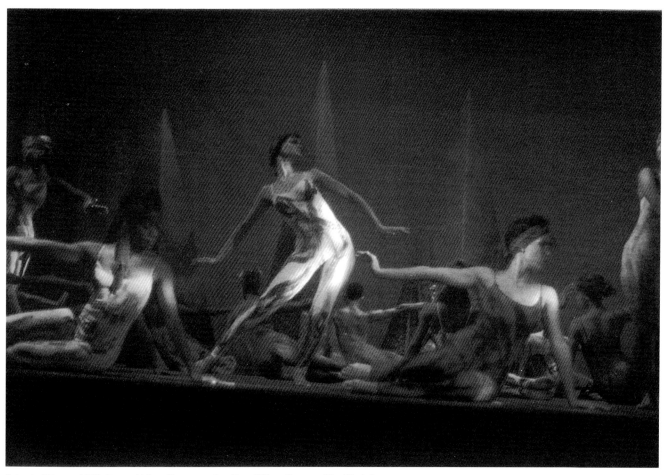

School of Dance, 1985 Dance: Voices Choreographer: Tony Wilson Dancers: The Workshop

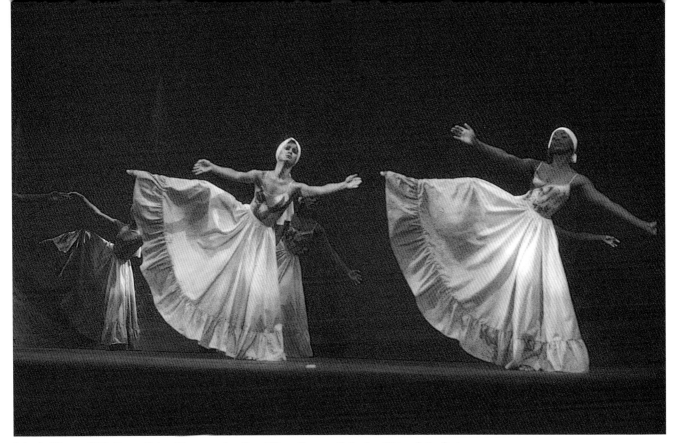

School of Dance, 1985 Dance: Voices Choreographer: Tony Wilson Dancers: Cathy Ann Gibbon & the Cast

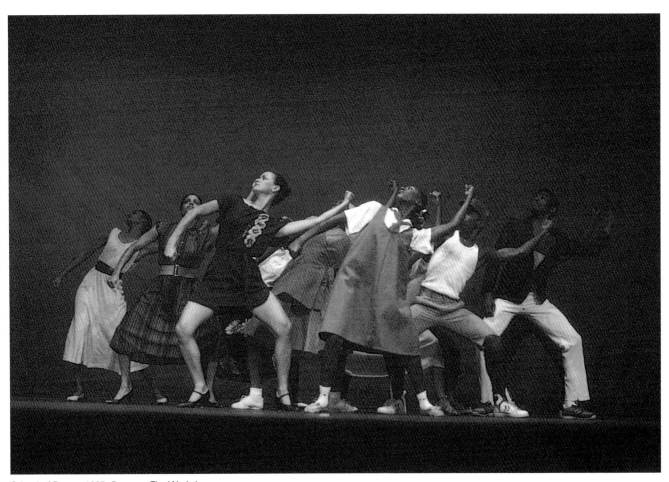

School of Dance, 1985 Dancers: The Workshop

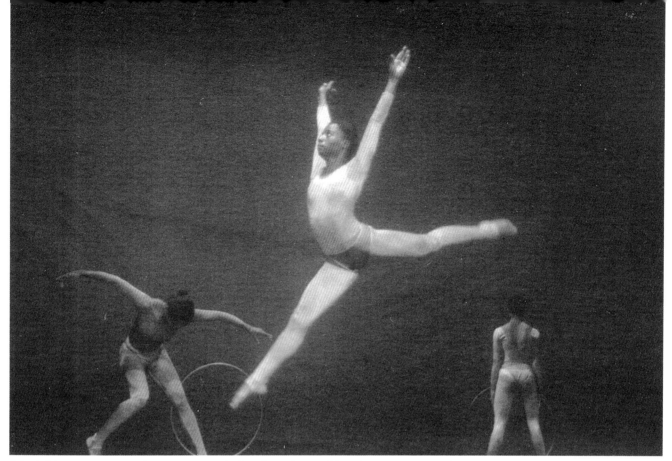

School of Dance, 1985 Dance: Trio Choreographer: Barbara Requa Dancers: Nicola Waite, Jacqui Logan, Staci-Lee Hassan-Fowles

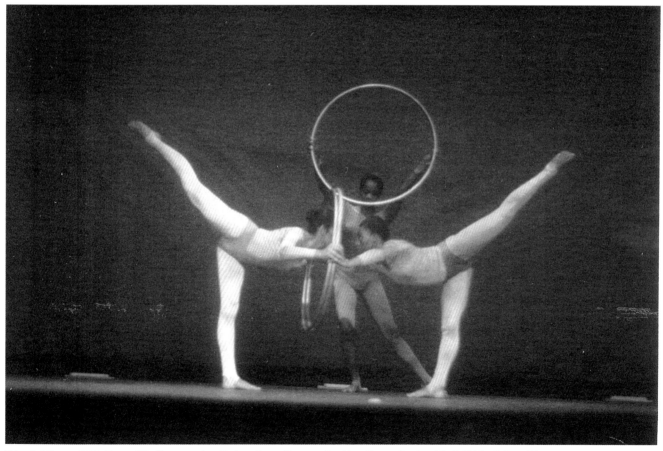

School of Dance, 1985 Dance: Trio Choreographer: Barbara Requa Dancers: Staci-Lee Hassan-Fowles, Nicola Waite & Jacqui Logan

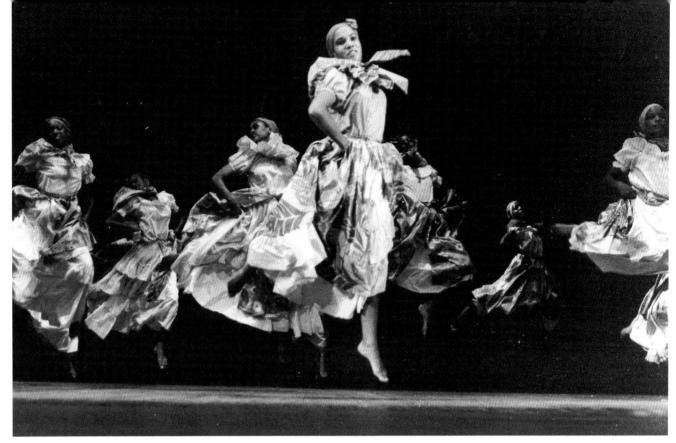

School of Dance, 1986 Dance: Belle Caribe Choreographer: Joseph Robinson Dancers: Clare Wilson & the Cast

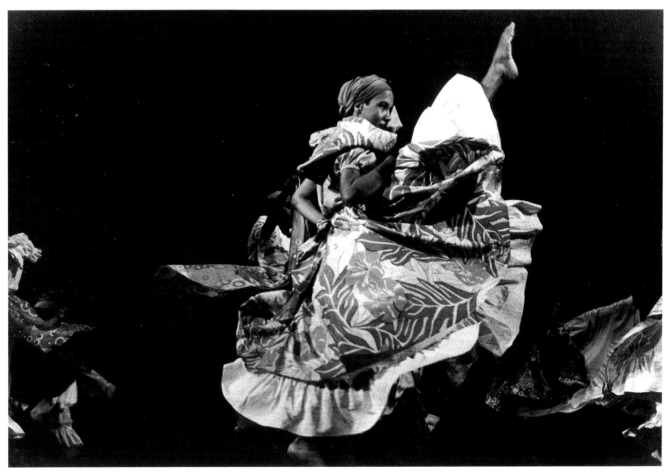

School of Dance, 1986 Dance: Belle Caribe Choreographer: Joseph Robinson Dancers: Clare Wilson & the Cast

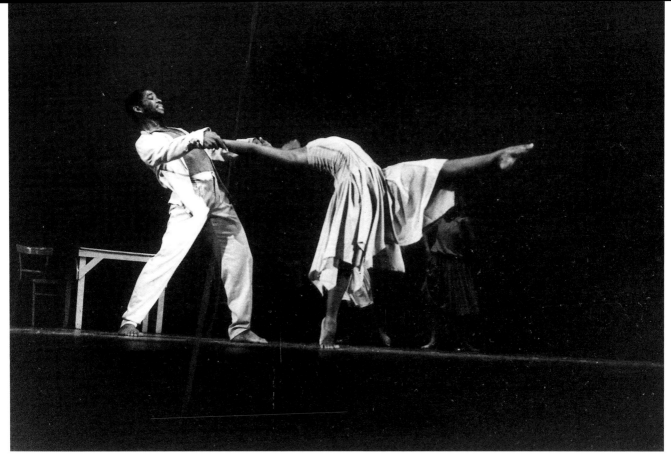

School of Dance, 1986 Dance: Love Games Choreographer: Barbara Requa Dancers: Joseph Robinson & Christine Rhone

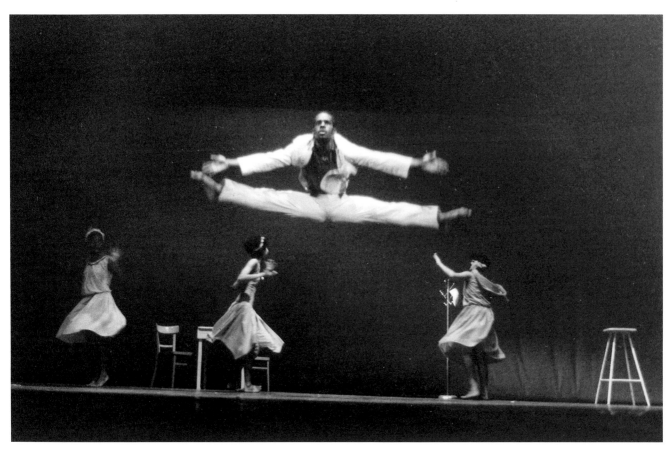

School of Dance, 1986 Dance: Love Games Choreographer: Barbara Requa Dancers: Dave Duncan, Jacqui Logan, Staci-Lee Hassan-Fowles & Clare Wilson

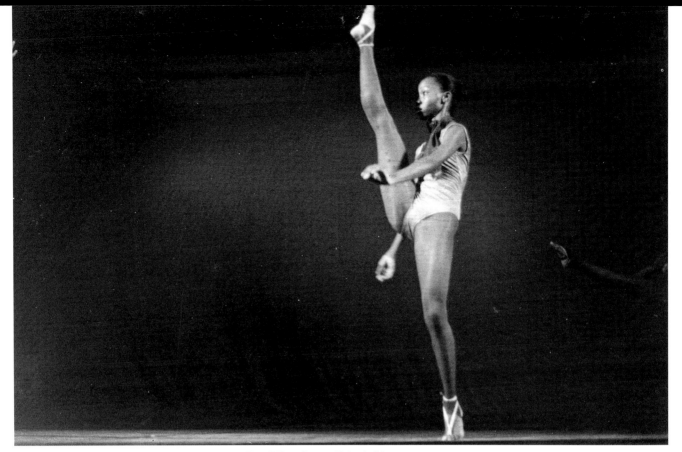

School of Dance, 1986 Dance: Phases Choreographer: Tony Wilson Dancer: Rolande Price

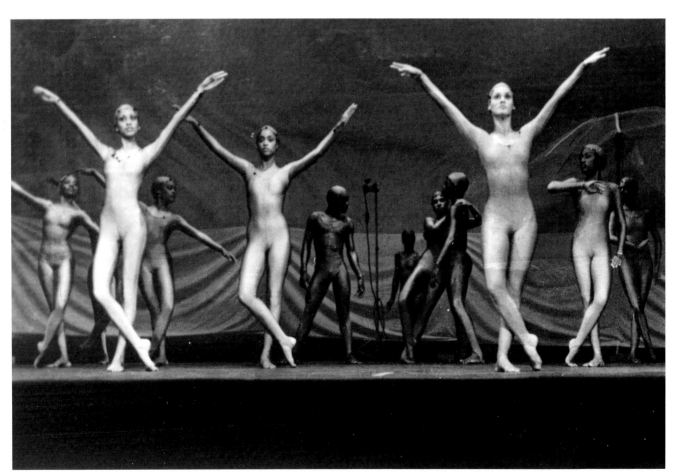

School of Dance, 1987 Dance: Collage Choreographer: Tony Wilson Dancers: Nicole Richards, Danielle Requa, Cathy-Ann Gibbon & the Cast

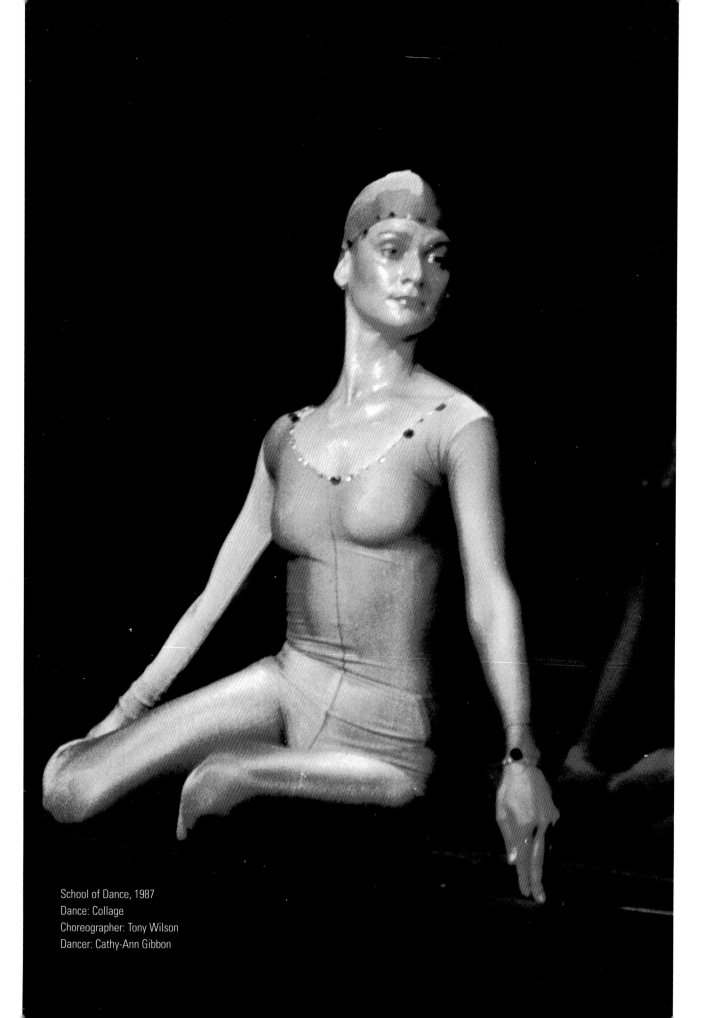

School of Dance, 1987
Dance: Collage
Choreographer: Tony Wilson
Dancer: Cathy-Ann Gibbon

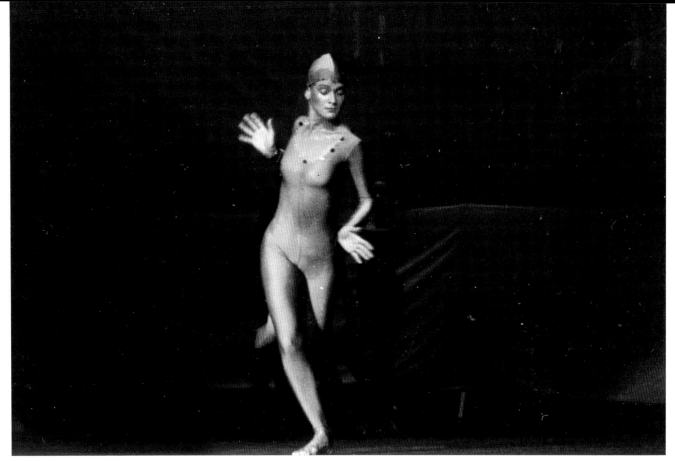

School of Dance, 1987 Dance: Collage Choreographer: Tony Wilson Dancer: Cathy-Ann Gibbon

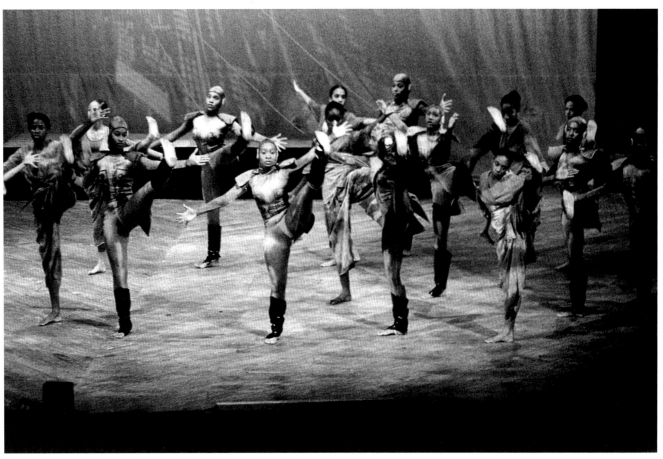

School of Dance, 1996 Dance: Circa 2002 Choreographer: Various Dancers: Cast of Junior Department (Seniors)

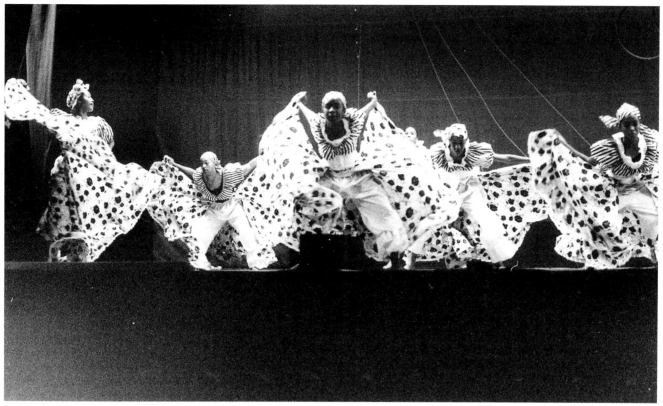

School of Dance, 1996 Dance: Circa 2002 Choreographer: Barbara Requa Dancers: Cast of Junior Department (Seniors)

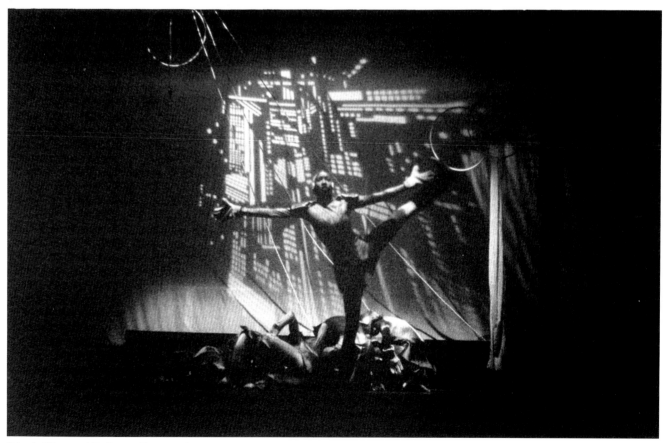

School of Dance, 1996 Dance: Circa 2002 Choreographer: Various Dancers: Tamara Noel & the Cast

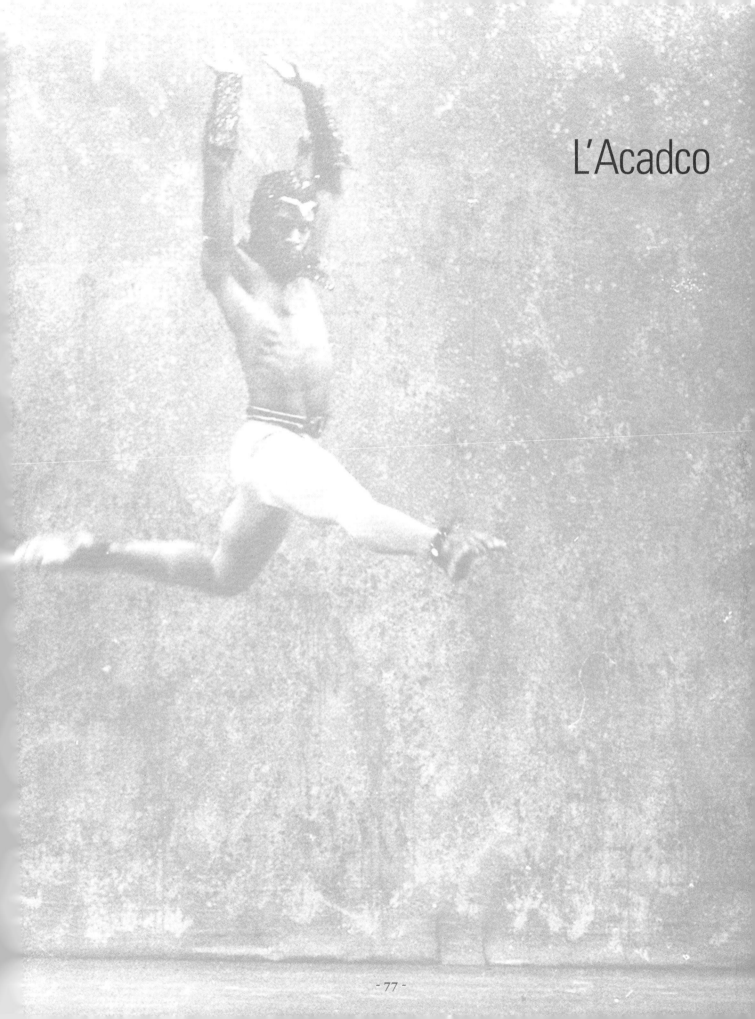

L'Acadco

L'Acadco – A United Caribbean Dance Force

In 1978, dancer/choreographer L'Antoinette Stines founded Miami's first, primarily black, dance company, L'Acadco. Returning to Jamaica in 1982, she continued to grow with her company and together they have become dynamic ambassadors for Jamaican culture and advocates for its sustained development and preservation.

Frequently participating in workshops and demonstrations to help educate younger dancers, these talented dancers represent the best in Caribbean talent. The company's membership has included dancers from Trinidad, Barbados, Guyana, The Bahamas and Suriname.

L'Acadco has toured overseas to promote Jamaican dance on the international market and has acted as a source for information on Caribbean-based modern dance techniques, as well as traditional dances. Internationally, L'Acadco has represented Jamaica in countries such as Mexico, Spain, France, Holland, Japan, England, Cuba, Trinidad and Ghana.

Today, the company is known as 'L'Acadco – A United Caribbean Dance Force' and is widely regarded as Jamaica's leading contemporary dance company. L'Acadco celebrated its 21st anniversary in 2004, and today it continues to raise the standard of dance in the Caribbean.

Electrifying audiences with their concerts and commercials, L'Acadco's freshness exudes from a revolutionary fusion and simultaneous presentation of rich Caribbean folklore with contemporary themes.

The distinctive training and choreography of L'Acadco is based on the L'Antech dance language created by L'Antoinette Stines. L'Acadco dancers are also exposed to international techniques on an ongoing basis: from training in Africa and Cuba, to employment in internationally-acclaimed companies, productions and institutions (such as Alvin Ailey, Garth Fagan, the London production of 'The Lion King' and 'Julliard').

L'Antoinette Stines, Artistic Director

…danced we our joy

our celebration our thanks

for that part of the journey

was rough beyond measure

so we danced our survival

and the pain and the pleasure

as too our vow

never never again

gaining strength

from those before us

for that journey ahead

now what we make is ours

the blame or the fame…

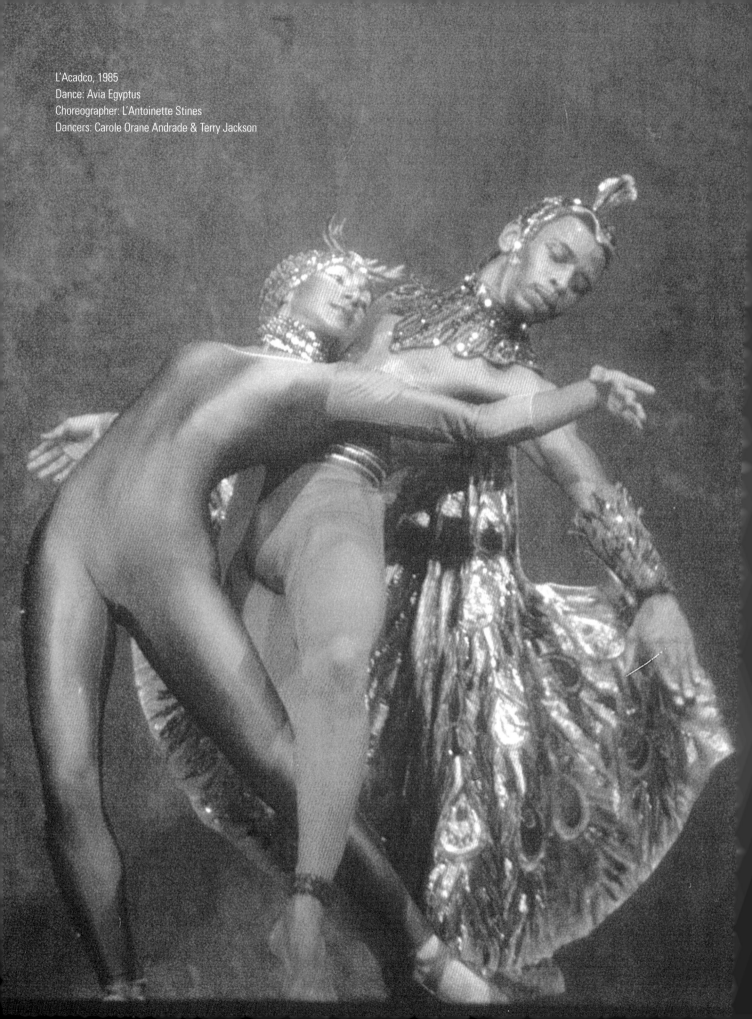

L'Acadco, 1985
Dance: Avia Egyptus
Choreographer: L'Antoinette Stines
Dancers: Carole Orane Andrade & Terry Jackson

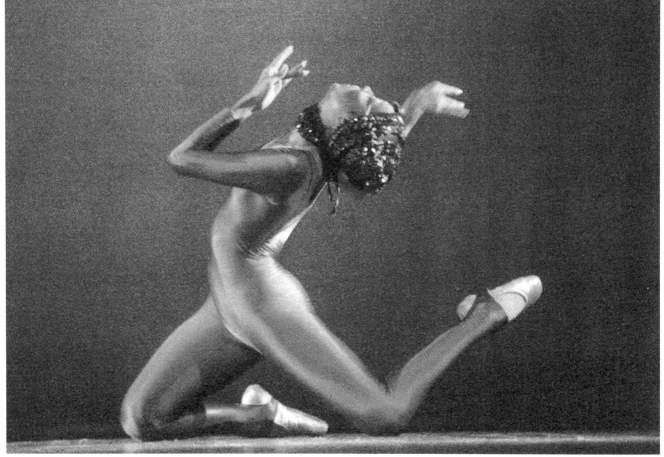

L'Acadco, 1985 Dance: Avia Egyptus Choreographer: L'Antoinette Stines Dancer: Desiree Ali

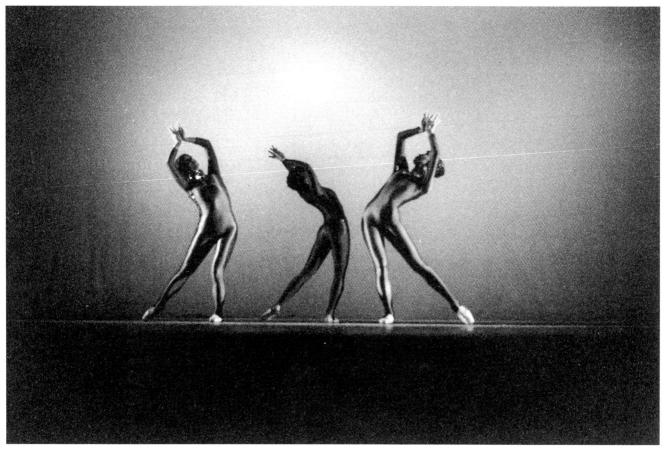

L'Acadco, 1985 Dance: Avia Egyptus Choreographer: L'Antoinette Stines Dancers: Tricia 'Yim' Johnston, Carole Orane Andrade & Desiree Ali

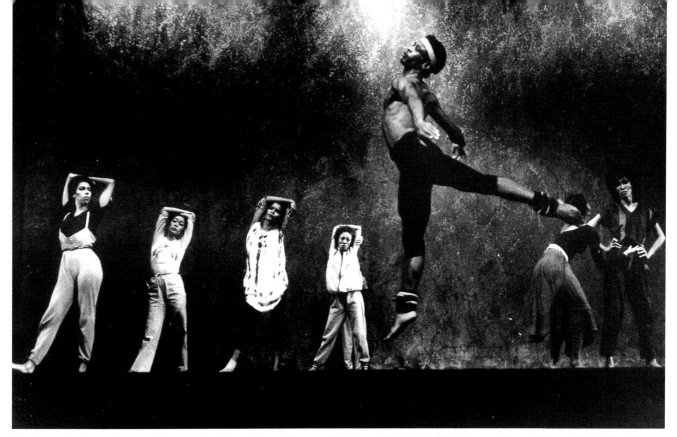

L'Acadco, 1985 Dance: Outamany Choreographer: Tommy Pinnock Dancers: Celia Jones-Hinds, Tricia 'Yim' Johnston, Rema Williams, Marie Minto, Terry Jackson, Carole Drane Andrade & Desiree Ali

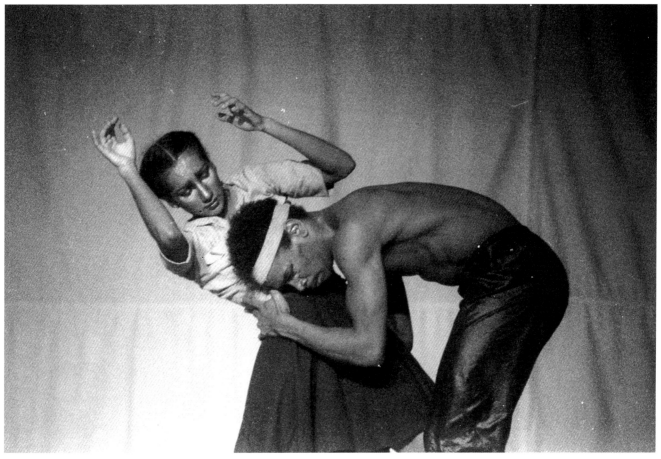

L'Acadco, 1985 Dance: Outamany Choreographer: Tommy Pinnock Dancers: Carole Orane Andrade & Terry Jackson (Cecil Charlton Hall, Mandeville)

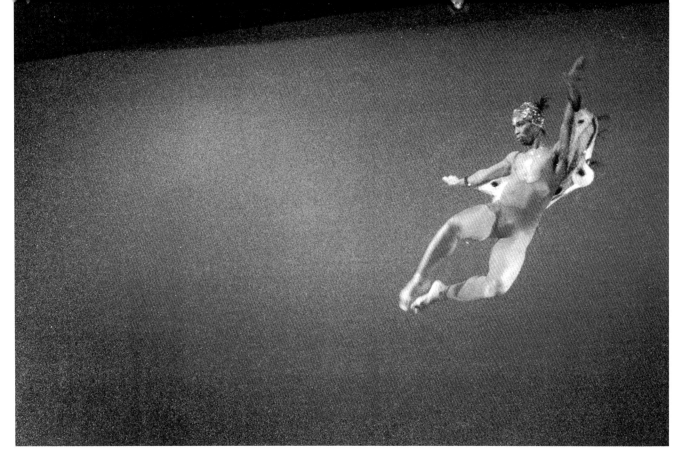

L'Acadco, 1985 Dance: Avia Egyptus Choreographer: L'Antoinette Stines Dancer: Terry Jackson

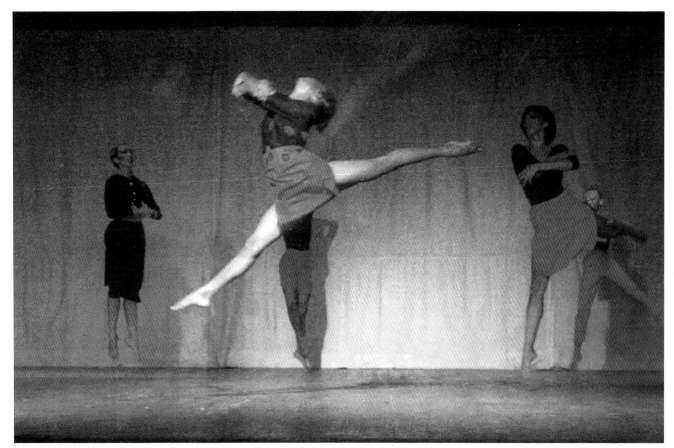

L'Acadco, 1985 Dance: High Choreographer: L'Antoinette Stines Dancers: Desiree Ali, Rema Williams, Celia Jones-Hinds & Marie Pinto
(Cecil Charlton Hall, Mandeville)

L'Acadco, 1985
Dance: Next
Choreographer: L'Antoinette Stines
Dancer: Carole Orane Andrade

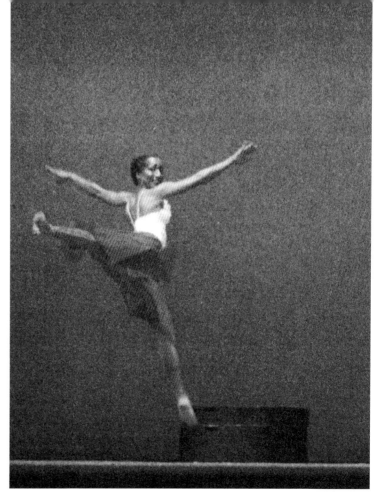

L'Acadco, 1985
Dance: High
Choreographer: L'Antoinette Stines
Dancers: Carole Orane Andrade & Terry Jackson

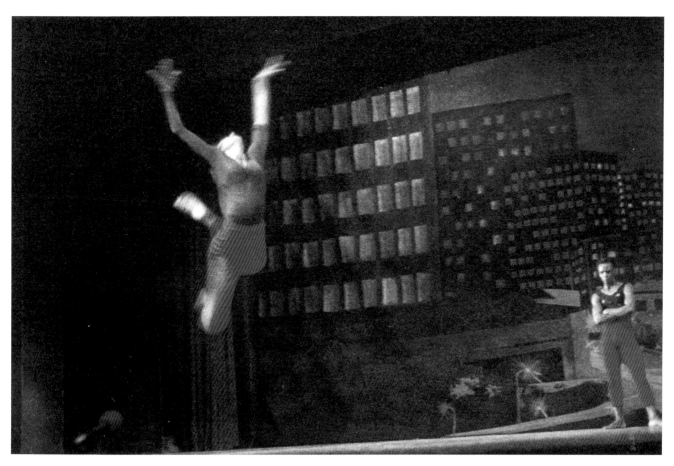

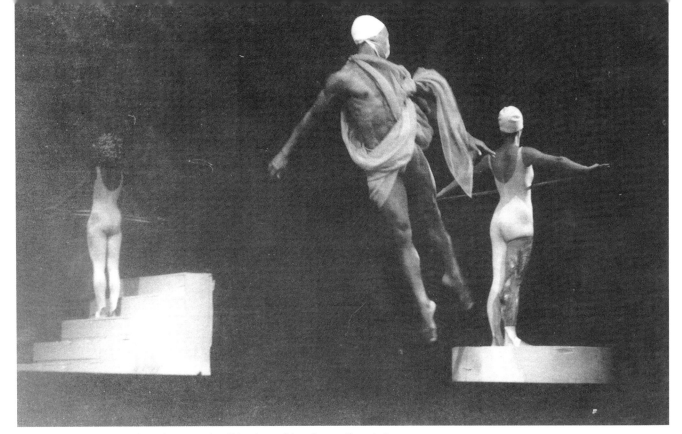

L'Acadco, 1985 Dance: Life Cycle Choreographer: L'Antoinette Stines Dancer: Terry Jackson

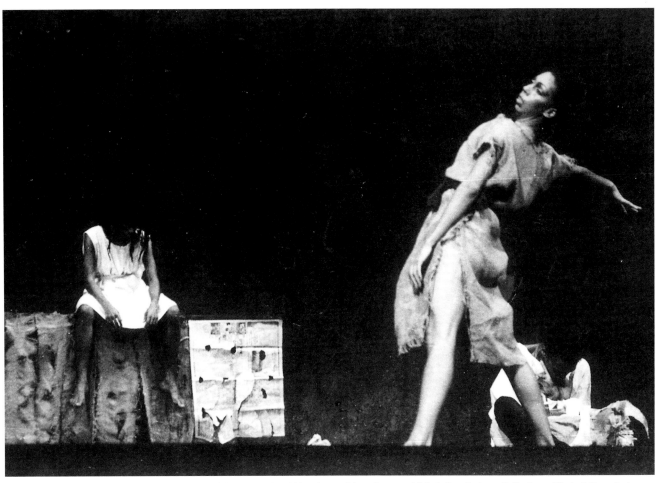

L'Acadco, 1985 Dance: Have You Ever Been There? Choreographer: L'Antoinette Stines Dancers: Melody Cunningham, Celia Jones-Hinds & Terry Jackson

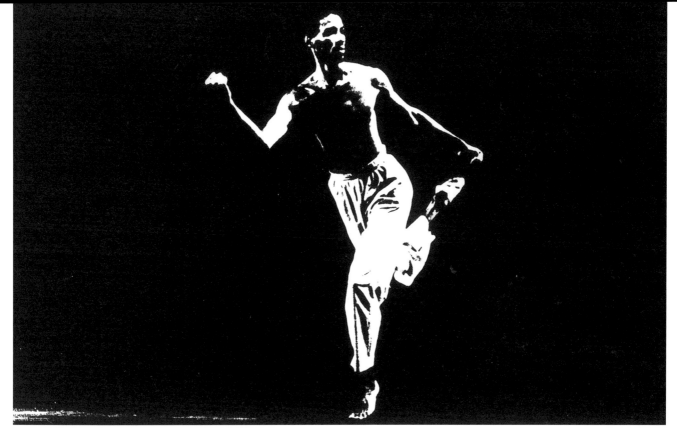

L'Acadco, 1986 Dance: Elements Choreographer: Howard Daley Dancer: Howard Daley

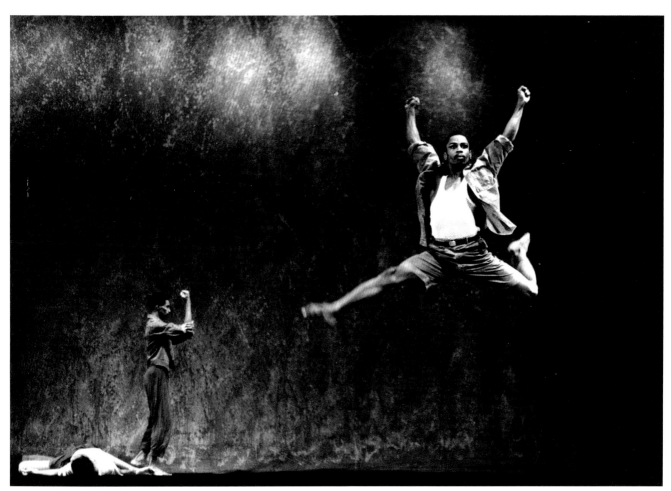

L'Acadco, 1986 Dance: Llow Mi Nuh Choreographer: Neville Black Dancer: Howard Daley & Terry Jackson

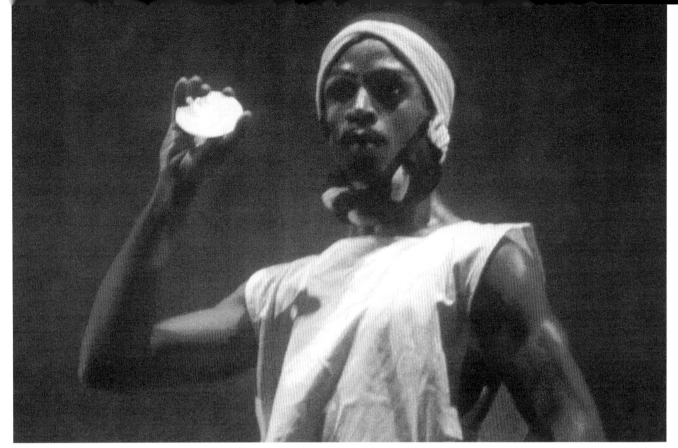

L'Acadco, 1986 Dance: Evolutia Choreographer: L'Antoinette Stines Dancer: Terry Jackson

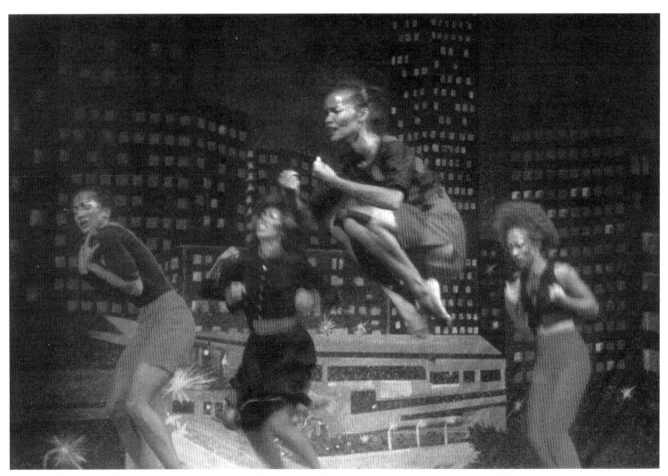

L'Acadco, 1986 Dance: High Choreographer: L'Antoinette Stines Dancers: Carole Orane Andrade, Desiree Ali, Rema Williams & Marie Minto

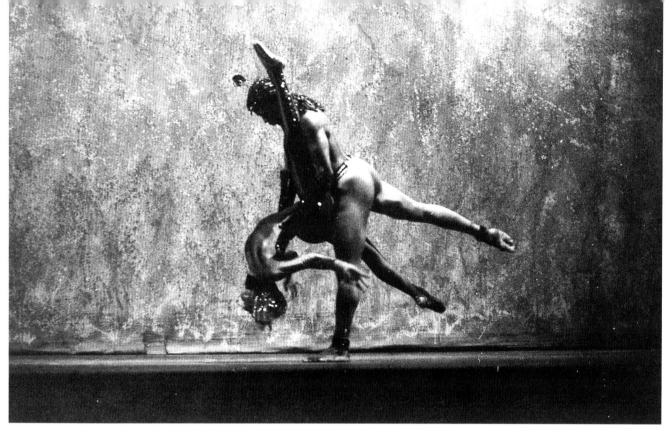

L'Acadco, 1986 Dance: Avia Egyptus Choreographer: L'Antoinette Stines Dancers: Carole Orane Andrade & Terry Jackson

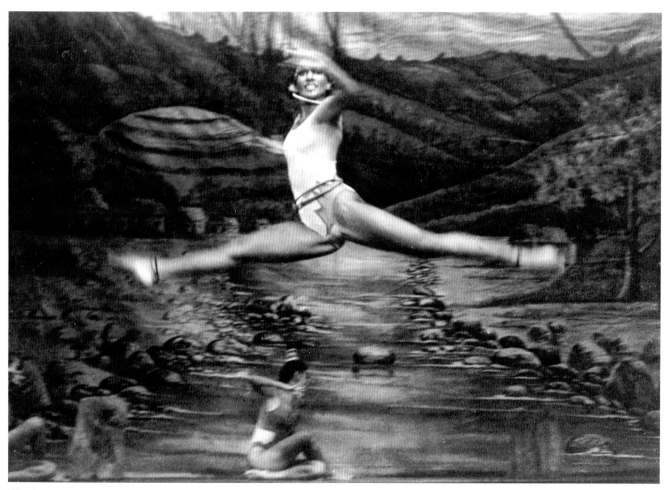

L'Acadco, 1986 Dance: Satta Choreographer: L'Antoinette Stines Dancer: Carole Orane Andrade

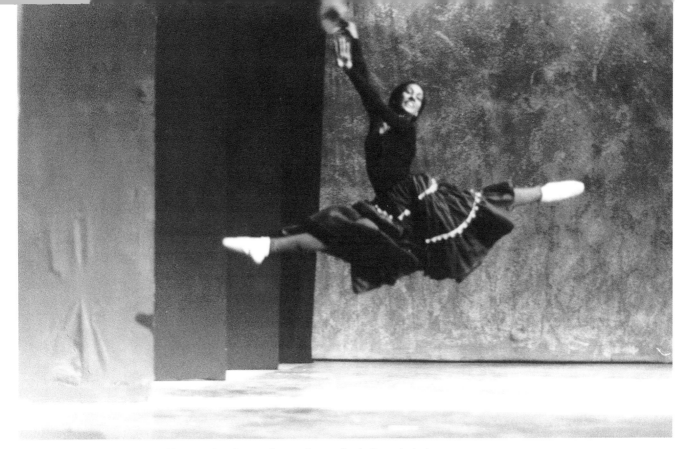

L'Acadco, 1986 Dance: Huapango Choreographer: Suzanne Iruegas Dancer: Carole Orane Andrade

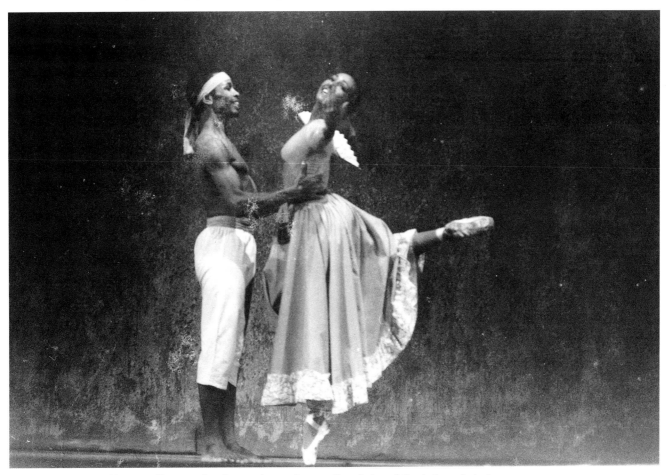

L'Acadco, 1986 Dance: Huapango Choreographer: Suzanne Iruegas Dancers: Terry Jackson & Carole Orane Andrade

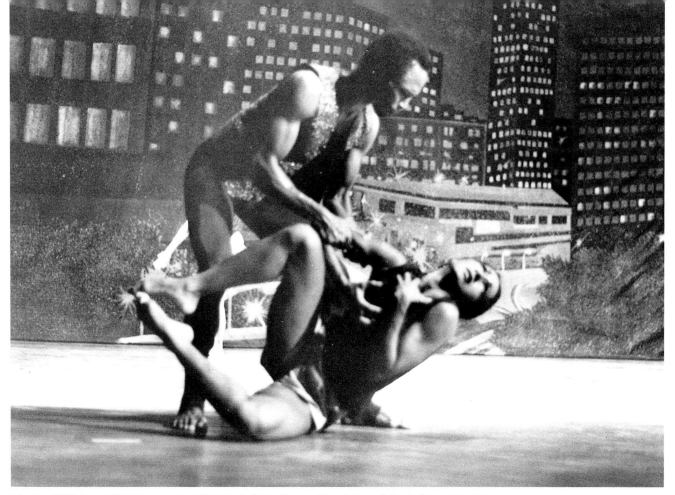

L'Acadco, 1986 Dance: High Choreographer: L'Antoinette Stines Dancers: Terry Jackson & Carole Orane Andrade

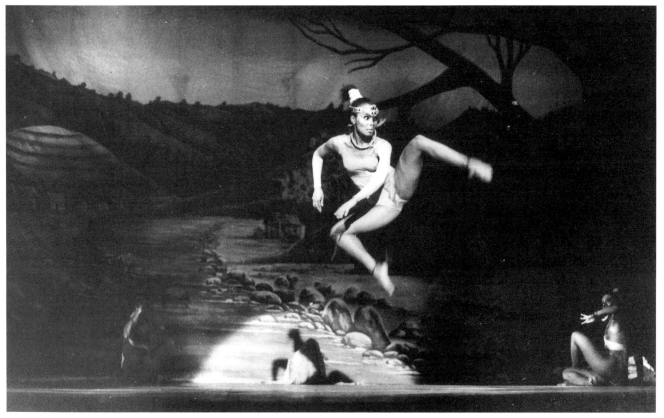

L'Acadco, 1989 Dance: Satta Choreographer: L'Antoinette Stines Dancer: Rema Williams

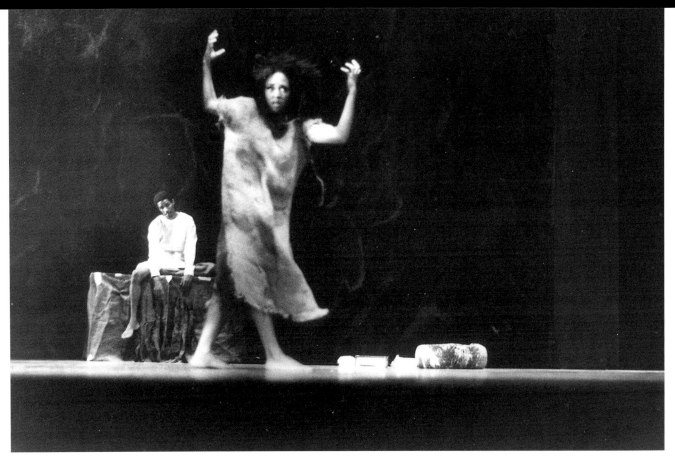

L'Acadco, 1989 Dance: Have You Ever Been There? Choreographer: L'Antoinette Stines Dancers: Howard Daley & Judy Tomlinson-Aikman

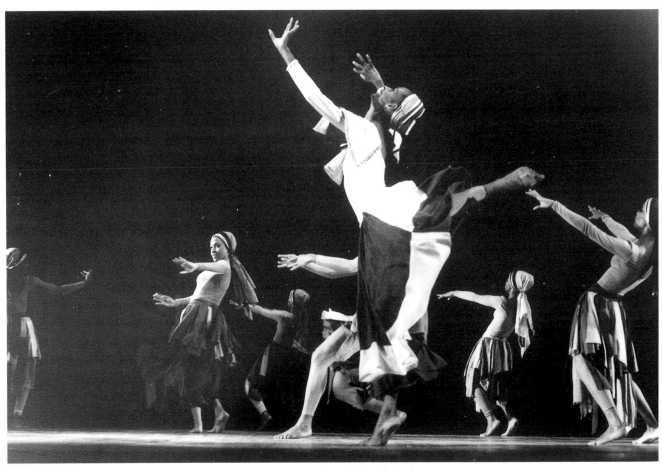

L'Acadco, 1989 Dance: Bingi Choreographer: L'Antoinette Stines Dancers: Patsy Ricketts & the Company

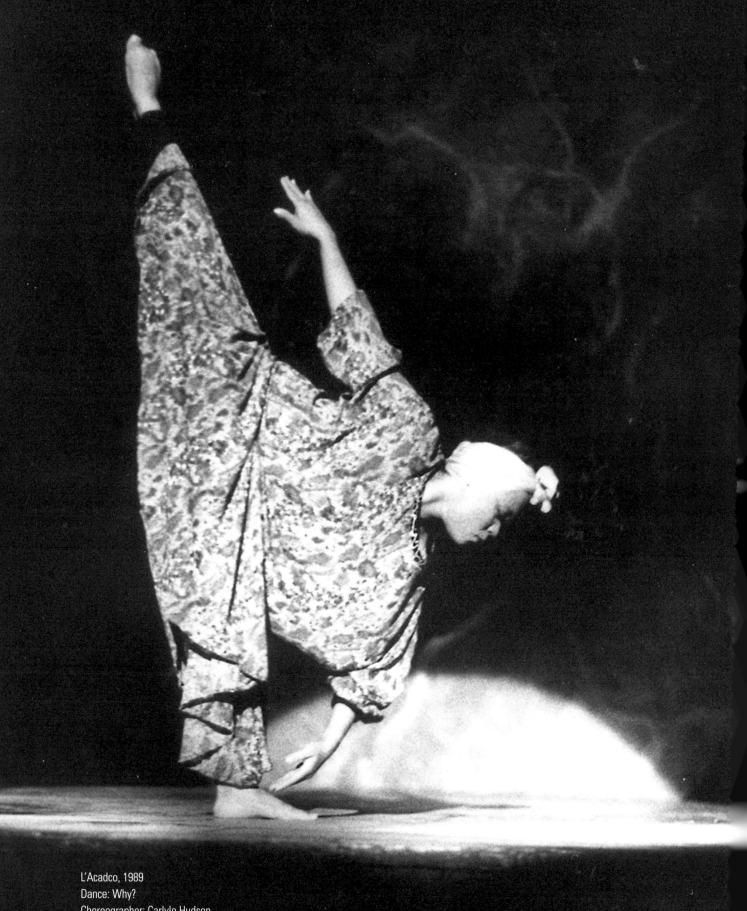

L'Acadco, 1989
Dance: Why?
Choreographer: Carlyle Hudson
Dancer: L'Antoinette Stines

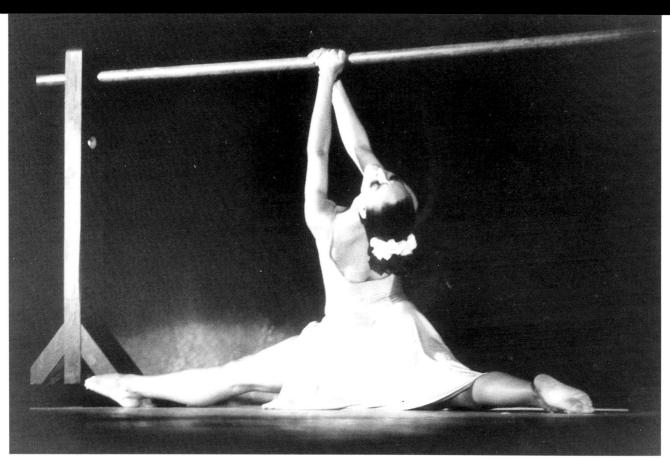

L'Acadco, 1989 Dance: Silent Partner Choreographer: Carole Orane Andrade Dancer: Judy Tomlinson-Aikman

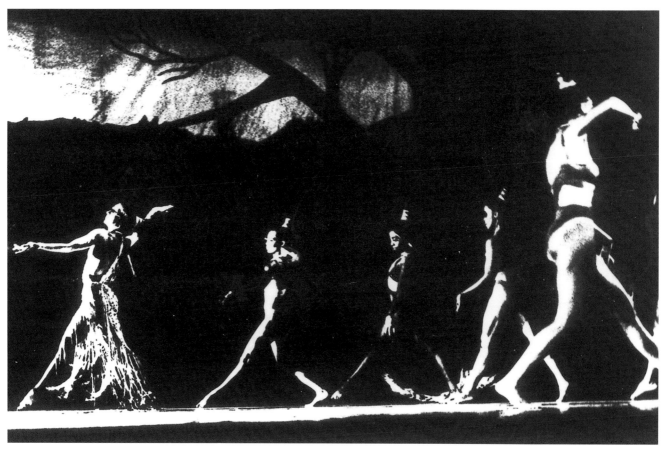

L'Acadco, 1989 Dance: Satta Choreographer: L'Antoinette Stines Dancers: Carole Orane Andrade, Rema Williams, Jacqui Logan, Judy Tomlinson-Aikman & Celia Jones-Hinds

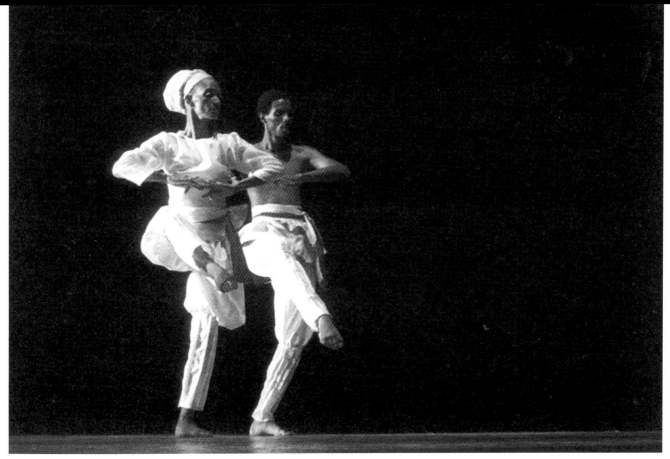

L'Acadco, 1989 Dance: Elements Choreographer: Howard Daley Dancers: Patsy Ricketts & Howard Daley

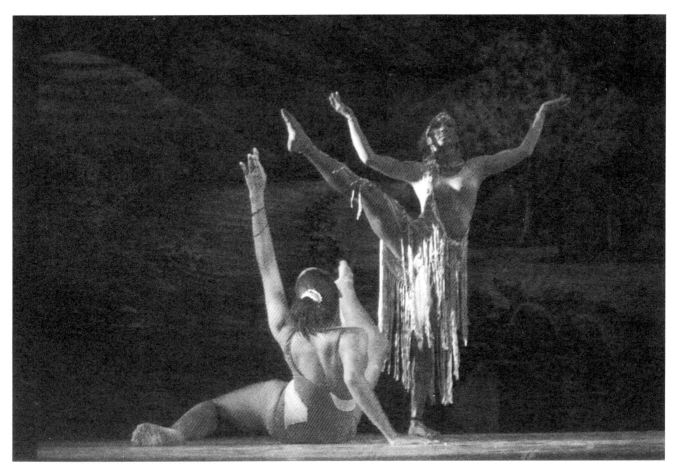

L'Acadco, 1989 Dance: Satta Choreographer: L'Antoinette Stines Dancers: Judy Tomlinson-Aikman & Carole Orane Andrade

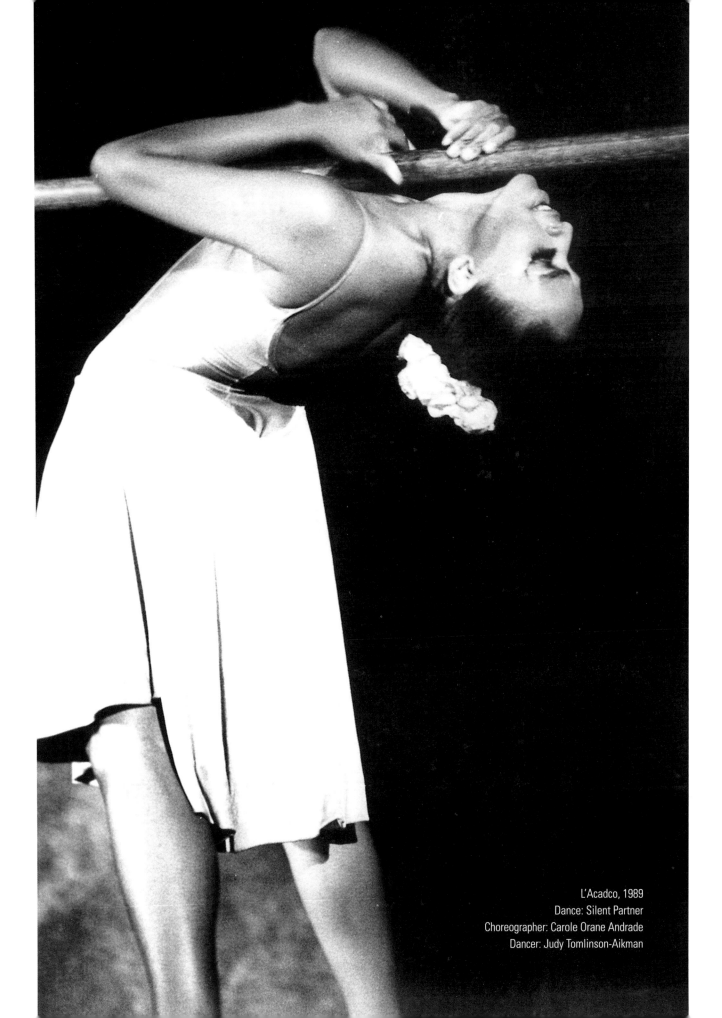

L'Acadco, 1989
Dance: Silent Partner
Choreographer: Carole Orane Andrade
Dancer: Judy Tomlinson-Aikman

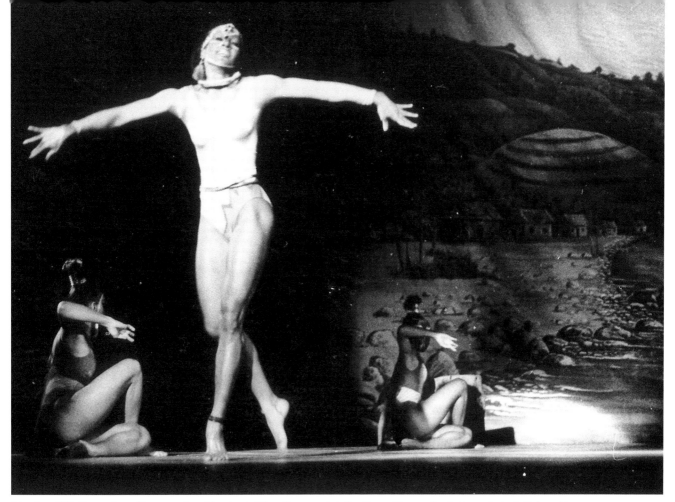

L'Acadco, 1989 Dance: Satta Choreographer: L'Antoinette Stines Dancers: Judy Tomlinson-Aikman, Carole Orane Andrade & Jacqui Logan

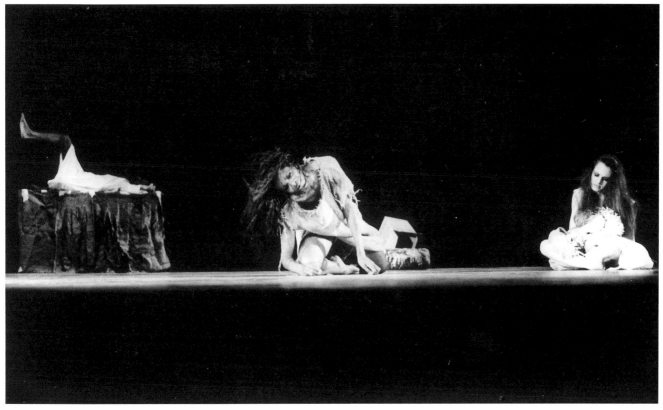

L'Acadco, 1989 Dance: Have You Ever Been There? Choreographer: L'Antoinette Stines Dancers: Howard Daley, Glenda Joseph-Dennis & Amy Laskin

L'Acadco, 1989 Dance: Elements Choreographer: Howard Daley Dancers: Patsy Ricketts & Howard Daley

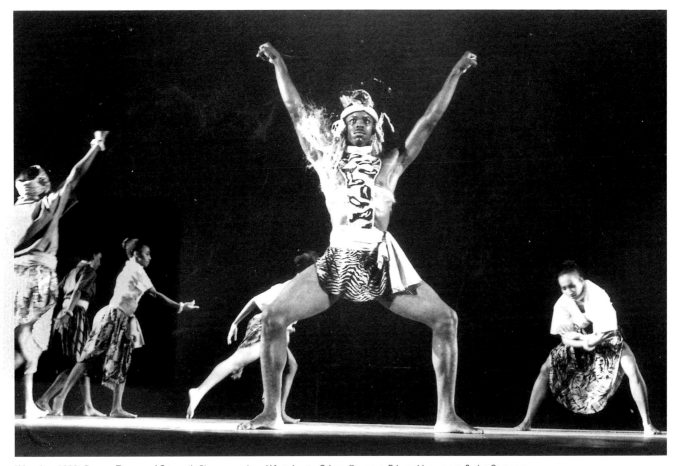

L'Acadco, 1989 Dance: Towers of Strength Choreographer: L'Antoinette Stines Dancers: Edward Lawrence & the Company

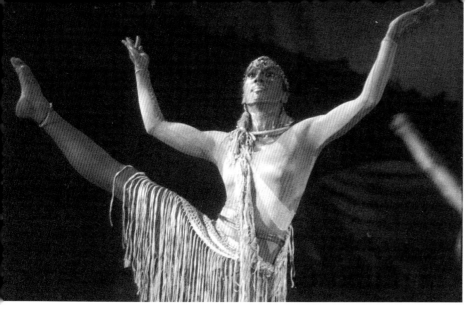

L'Acadco, 1989
Dance: Satta
Choreographer: L'Antoinette Stines
Dancer: Carole Orane Andrade

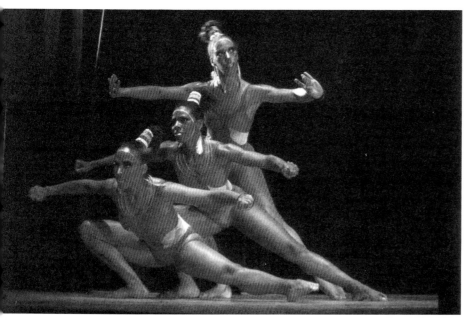

L'Acadco, 1989
Dance: Satta
Choreographer: L'Antoinette Stines
Dancers: Judy Tomlinson-Aikman,
Glenda Joseph-Dennis & Celia Jones-Hinds

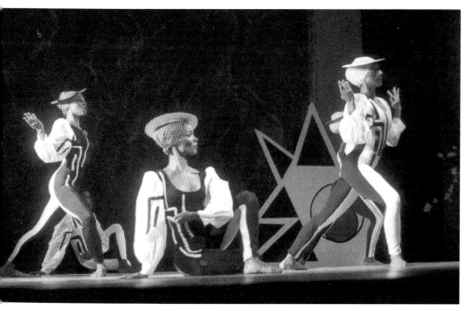

L'Acadco, 1989
Dance: Syncrisis
Choreographer: L'Antoinette Stines
Dancers: Judy Tomlinson-Aikman, Rema Williams &
Carole Orane Andrade

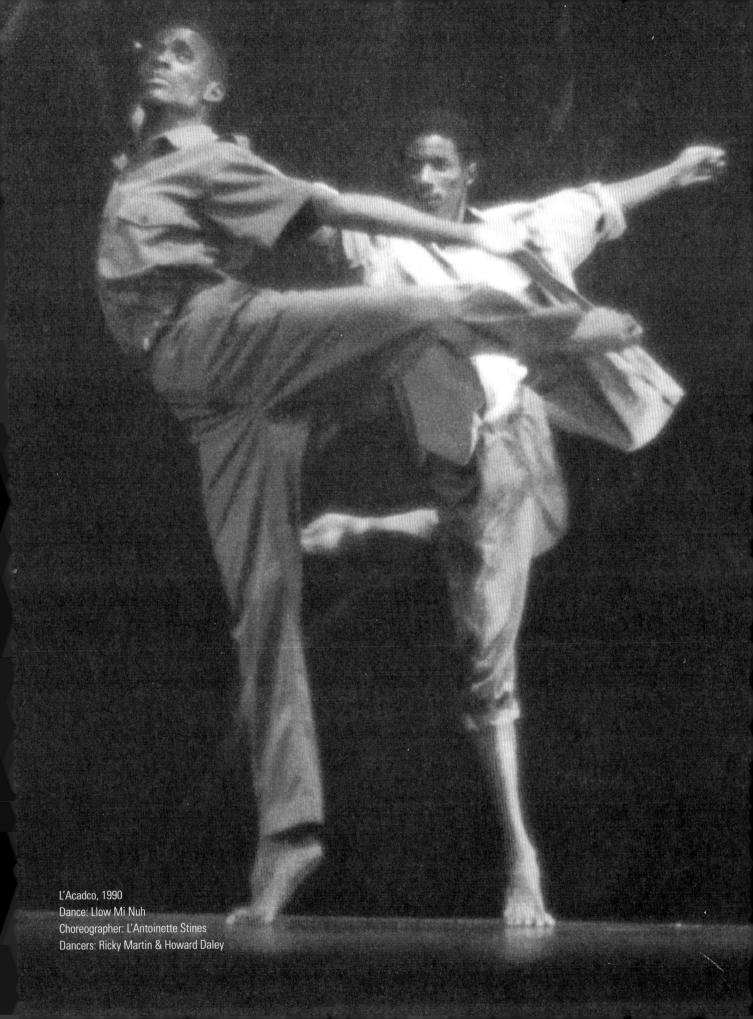

L'Acadco, 1990
Dance: Llow Mi Nuh
Choreographer: L'Antoinette Stines
Dancers: Ricky Martin & Howard Daley

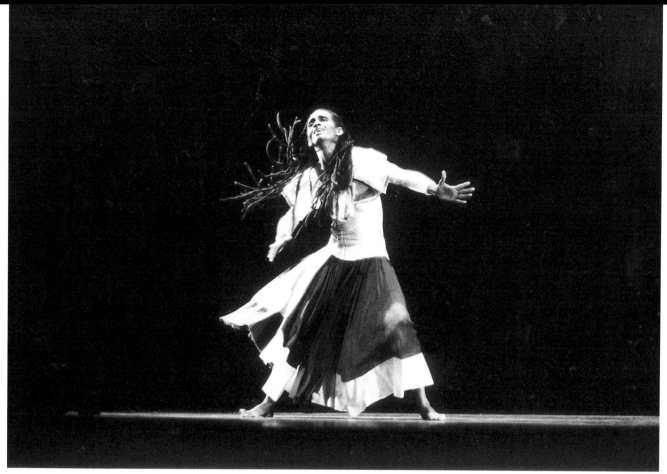

L'Acadco, 1990 Dance: Bingi Choreographer: L'Antoinette Stines Dancer: Patsy Ricketts

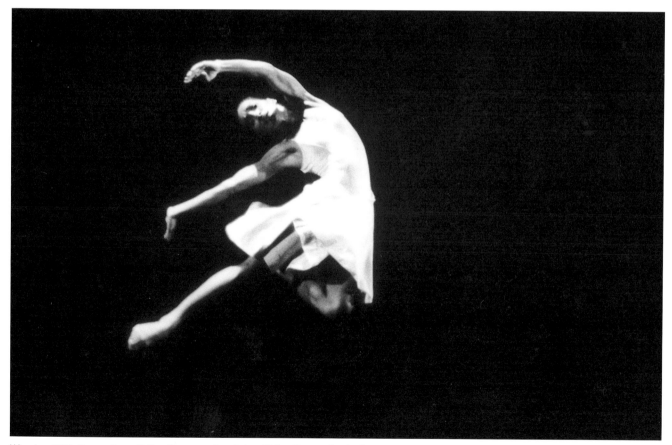

L'Acadco, 1990 Dance: Down To You Choreographer: Robert Bisbee Dancer: Carole Orane Andrade

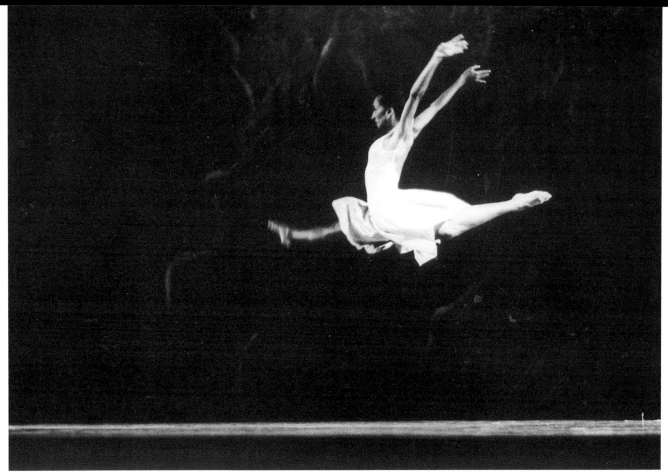

L'Acadco, 1990 Dance: Down To You Choreographer: Robert Bisbee Dancer: Carole Orane Andrade

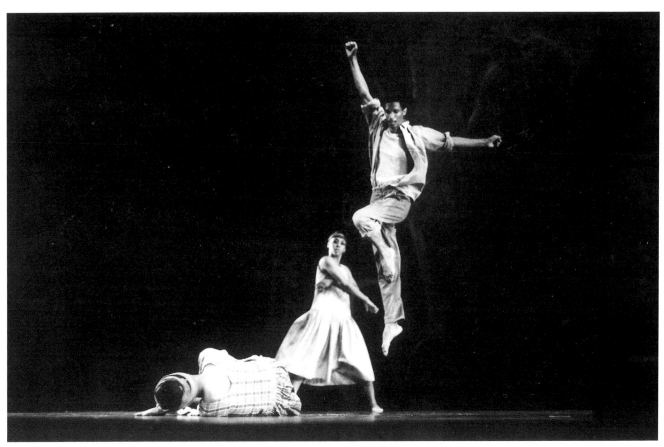

L'Acadco, 1990 Dance: Llow Mi Nuh Choreographer: L'Antoinette Stines Dancers: Jacqui Logan, Judy Tomlinson-Aikman & Howard Daley

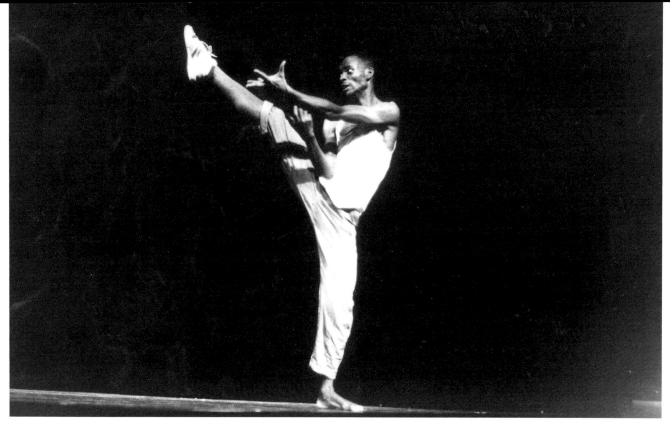

L'Acadco, 1990 Dance: Unseen Walls Choreographer: L'Antoinette Stines Dancer: Ricky Martin

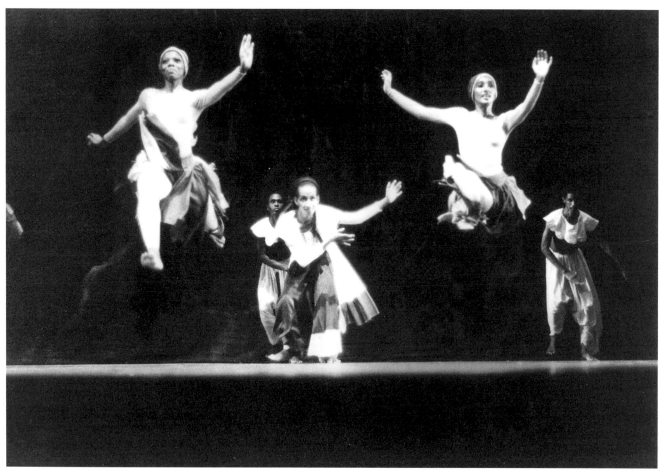

L'Acadco, 1990 Dance: Bingi Choreographer: L'Antoinette Stines Dancers: Glenda Joseph-Dennis, Glenmore Reed, Patsy Ricketts, Carole Orane Andrade & Howard Daley

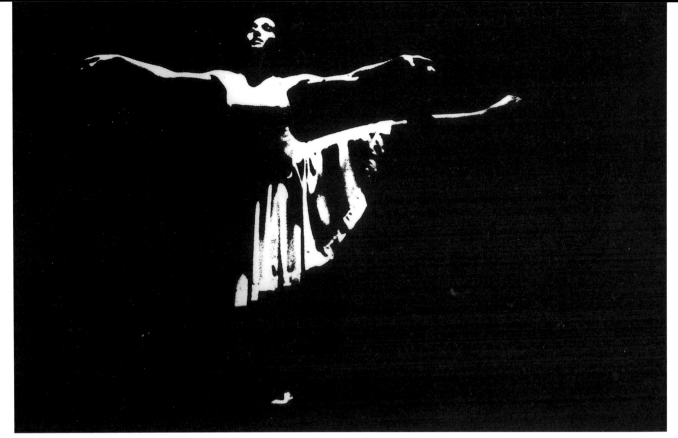

L'Acadco, 1990 Dance: Down to You Choreographer: Robert Bisbee Dancer: Carole Orane Andrade

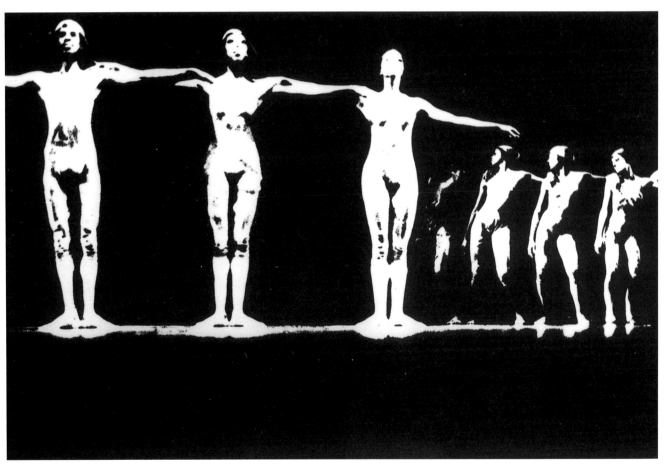

L'Acadco, 1990 Dance: Noisy Art Choreographer: Terry Jackson Dancers: Howard Daley, Celia Jones-Hinds, Judy Tomlinson-Aikman, Ricky Marti8n, Glenda Joseph-Dennis, Lisa Soares-Officer & Amy Laskin

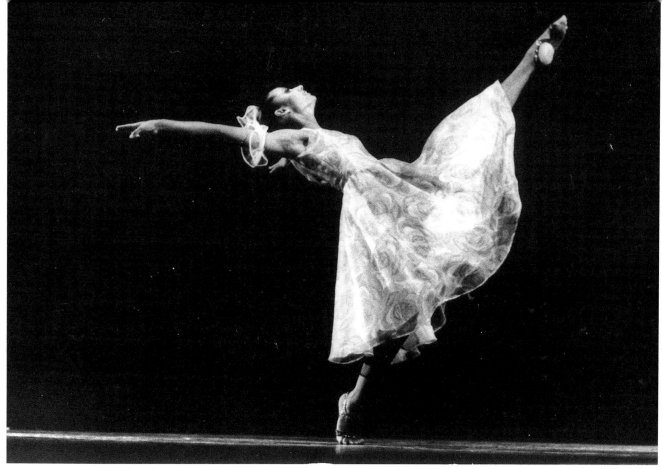

L'Acadco, 1990 Dance: Shades Choreographer: Neville Black Dancer: Lisa Soares-Officer

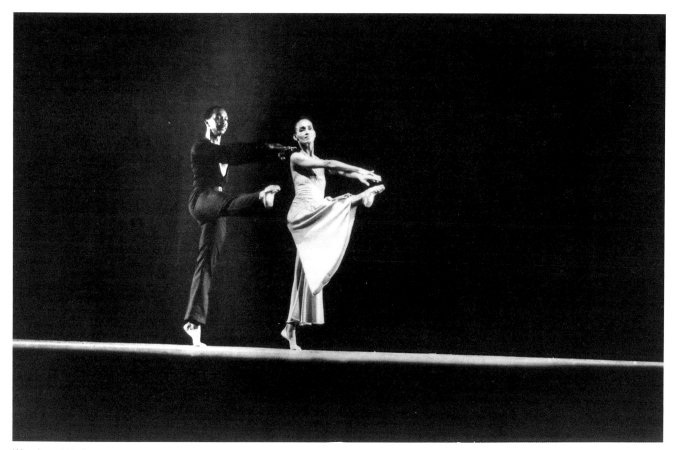

L'Acadco, 1990 Dance: Many Rivers to Cross Choreographer: Rex Nettleford Dancers: Barry Montcriffe & Patsy Ricketts

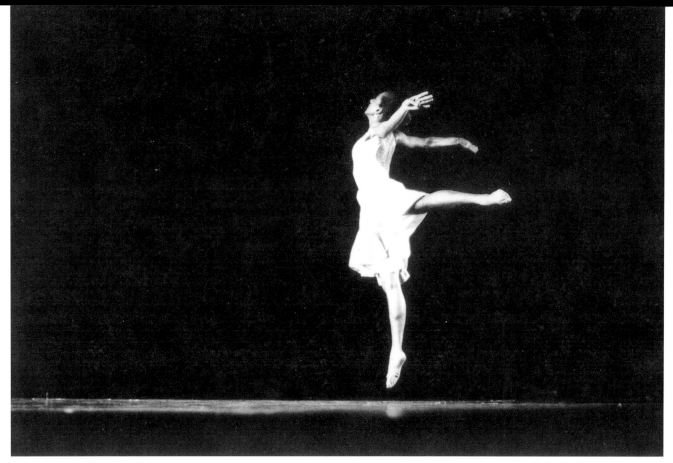

L'Acadco, 1990 Dance: Down to You Choreographer: Robert Bisbee Dancer: Carole Orane Andrade

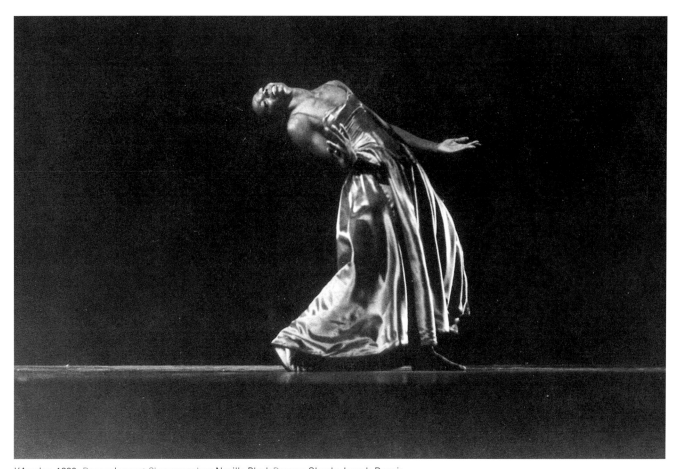

L'Acadco, 1990 Dance: Lament Choreographer: Neville Black Dancer: Glenda Joseph-Dennis

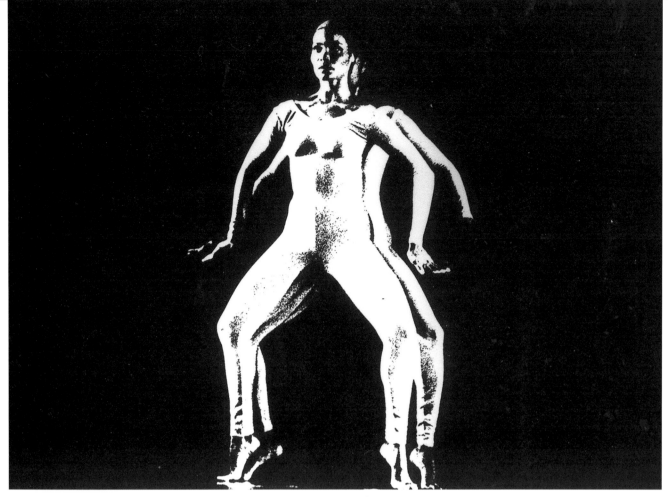

L'Acadco, 1992 Dance: Alpha Choreographer: Gene Carson Dancers: Rema Williams & Clara Reyes

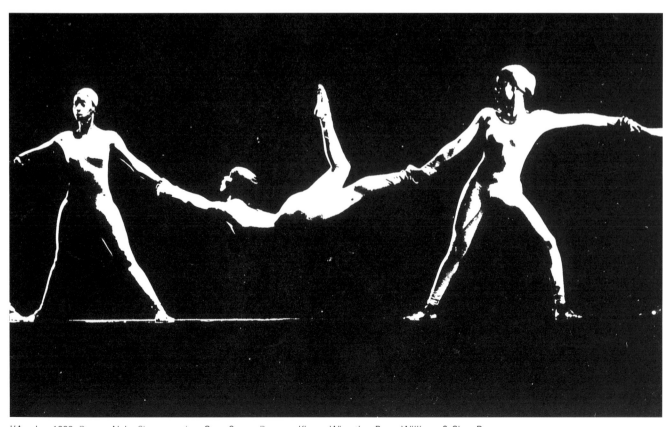

L'Acadco, 1992 Dance: Alpha Choreographer: Gene Carson Dancers: Khama Wheatley, Rema Williams & Clara Reyes

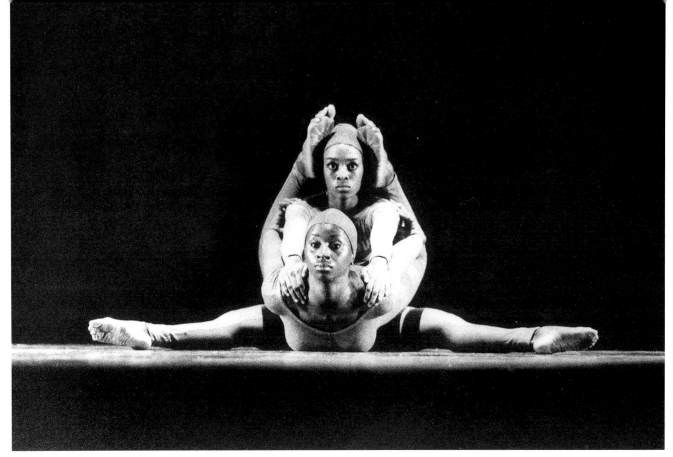

L'Acadco, 1992 Dance: Alpha Choreographer: Gene Carson Dancers: Khama Wheatley & Lisa Ogilvie

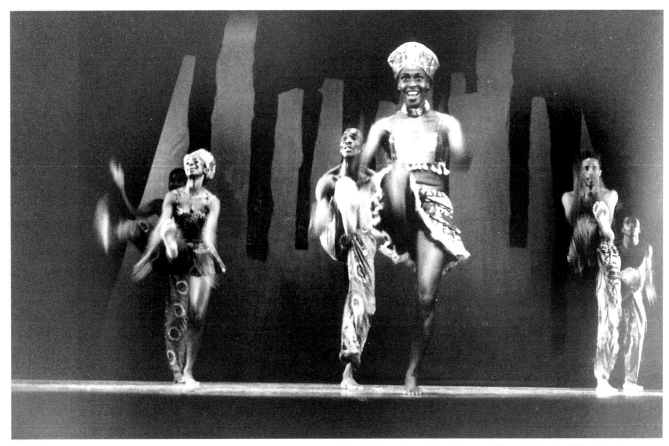

L'Acadco, 1992 Dance: Amathagazelo Choreographers: Clara Reyes, Howard Daley & L'Antoinette Stines Dancers: Khama Wheatley, Ricky Martin, Clara Reyes, Howard Daley & Glenmore 'Wayne' Reed

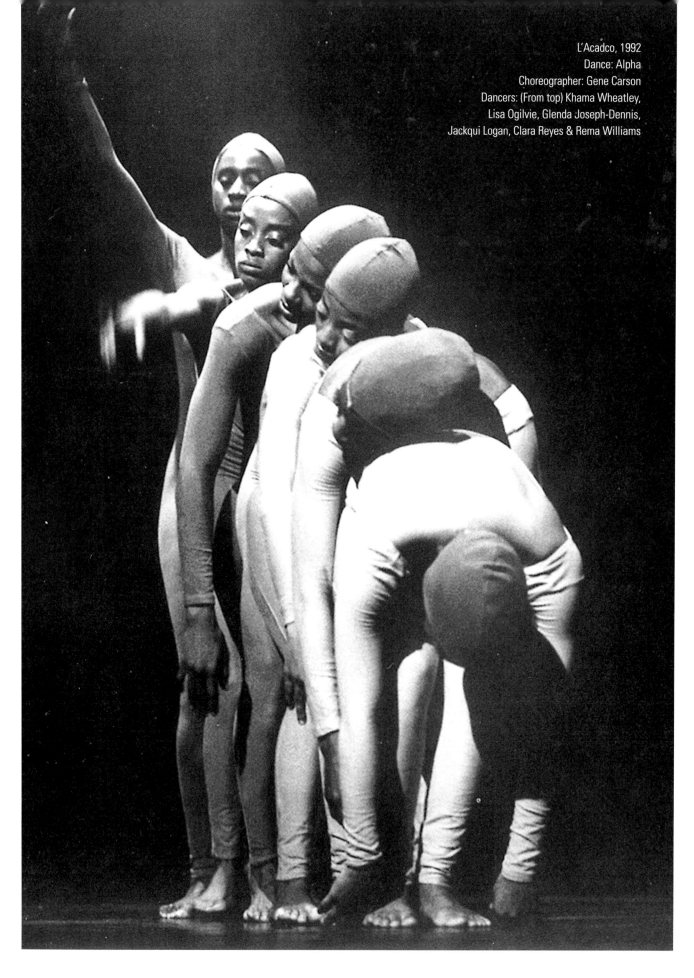

L'Acadco, 1992
Dance: Alpha
Choreographer: Gene Carson
Dancers: (From top) Khama Wheatley,
Lisa Ogilvie, Glenda Joseph-Dennis,
Jackqui Logan, Clara Reyes & Rema Williams

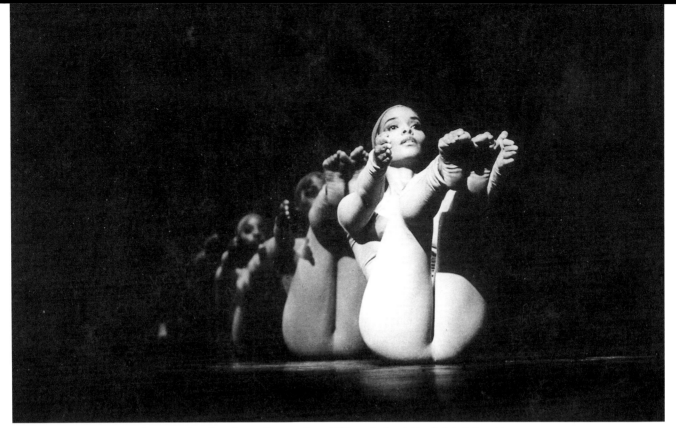

L'Acadco, 1992 Dance: Alpha Choreographer: Gene Carson Dancers: Rema Williams (in front), Lisa Ogilvie & Jacqui Logan

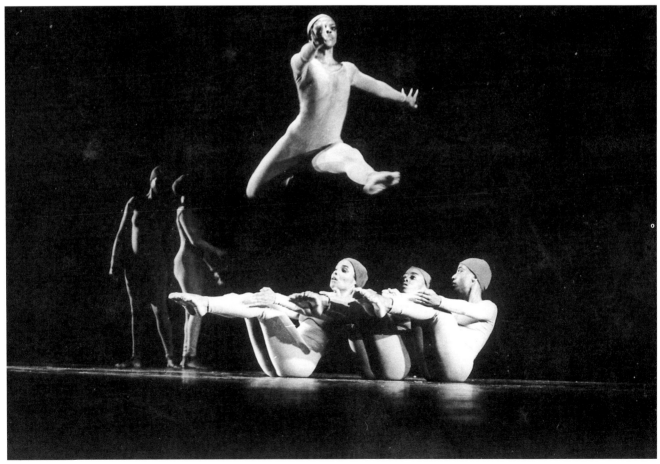

L'Acadco, 1992 Dance: Alpha Choreographer: Gene Carson Dancers: Khama Wheatley, Clara Reyes, Glenda Joseph-Dennis (in air), Rema Williams, Lisa Ogilvie & Jacqui Logan

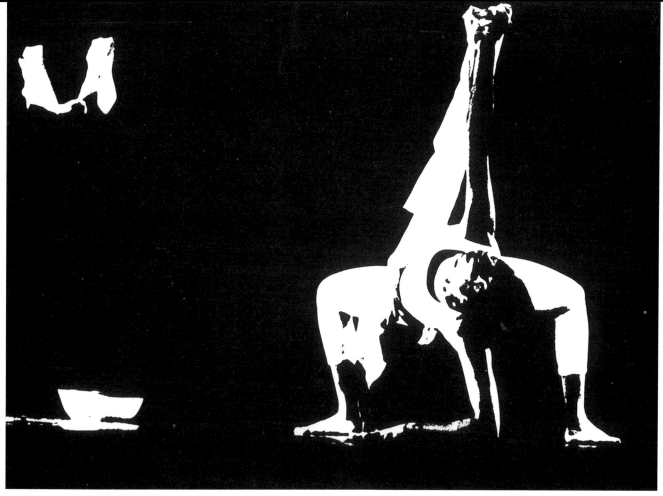

L'Acadco, 1992 Dance: Tribulation Choreographer: L'Antoinette Stines Dancer: Rema Williams

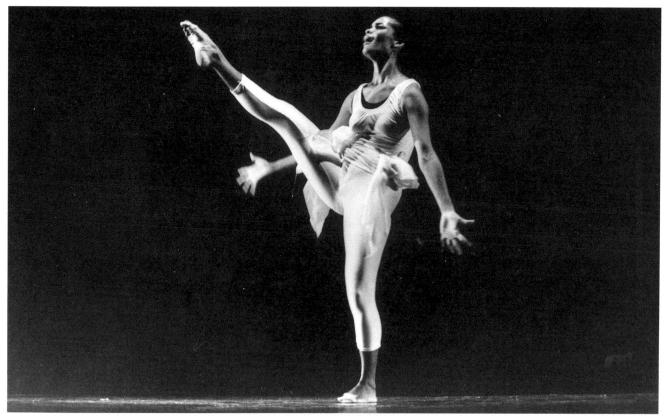

L'Acadco, 1992 Dance: Tribulation Choreographer: L'Antoinette Stines Dancer: Rema Williams

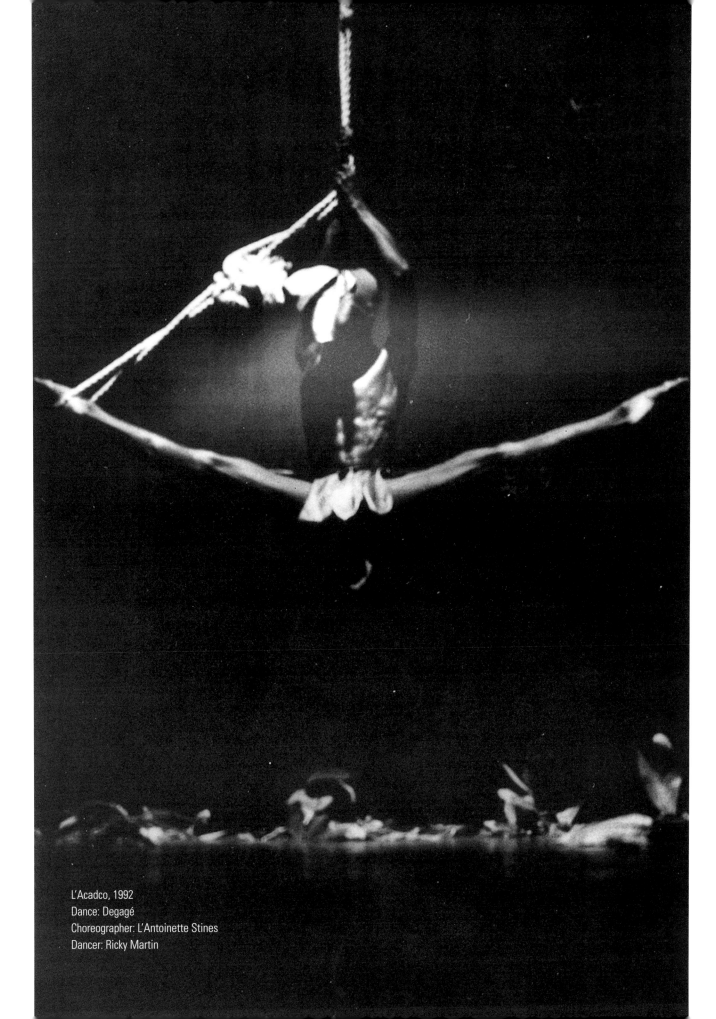

L'Acadco, 1992
Dance: Degagé
Choreographer: L'Antoinette Stines
Dancer: Ricky Martin

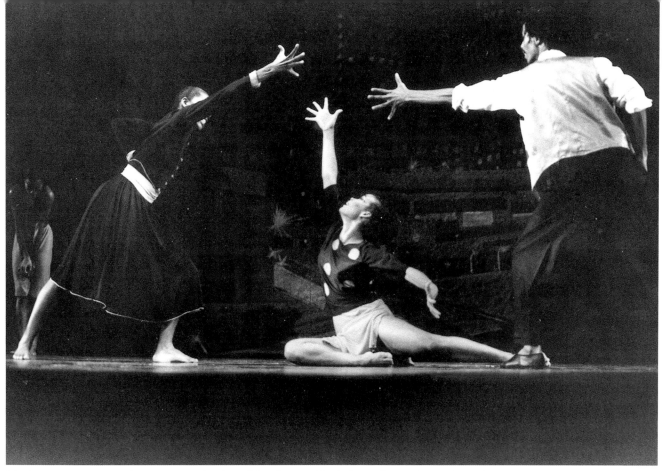

L'Acadco, 1992 Dance: High Choreographer: L'Antoinette Stines Dancers: Glenda Joseph-Dennis, Rema Williams & Howard Daley

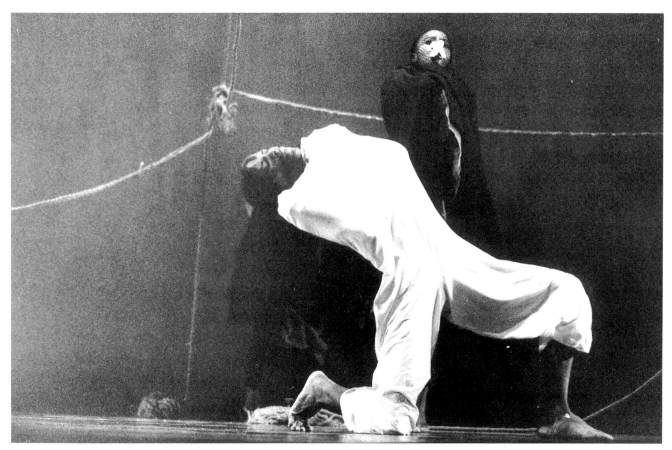

L'Acadco, 1992 Dance: Libertad Choreographer: L'Antoinette Stines Dancers: Howard Daley & Lisa Ogilvie

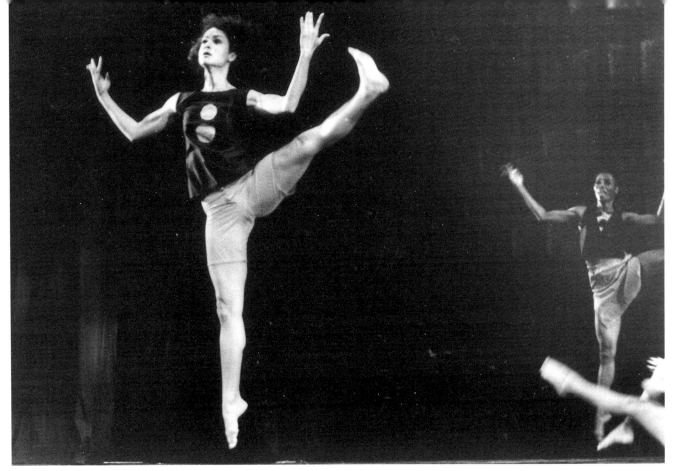

L'Acadco, 1992 Dance: High Choreographer: L'Antoinette Stines Dancer: Cathy Ann Gibbon

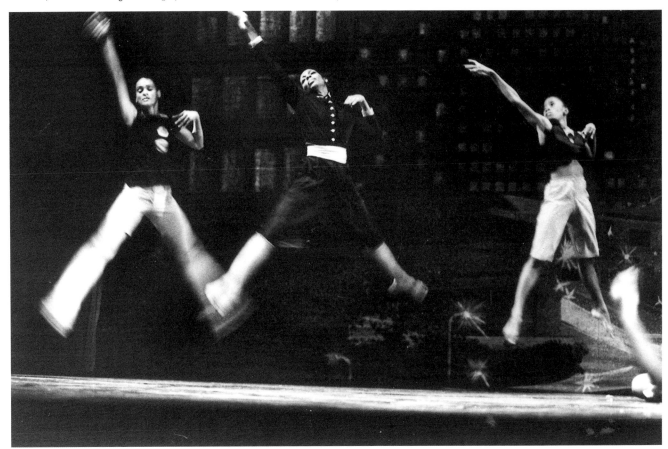

L'Acadco, 1992 Dance: High Choreographer: L'Antoinette Stines Dancers: Cathy Ann Gibbon, Glenda Joseph-Dennis & Lisa Ogilvie

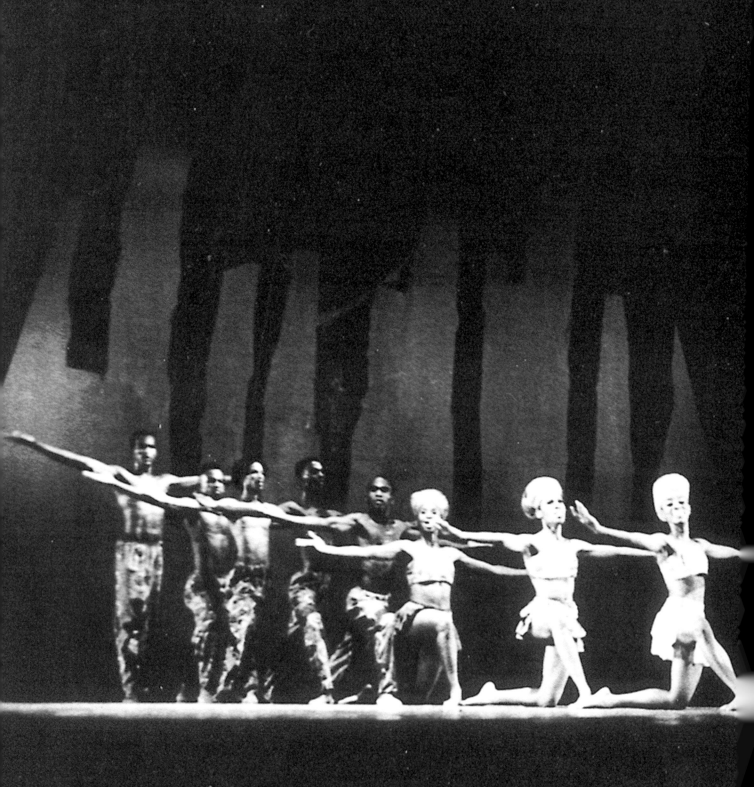

L'Acadco, 1992
Dance: Amathagazelo
Choreographers: Clara Reyes, Howard Daley & L'Antoinette Stines
Dancers: The Company

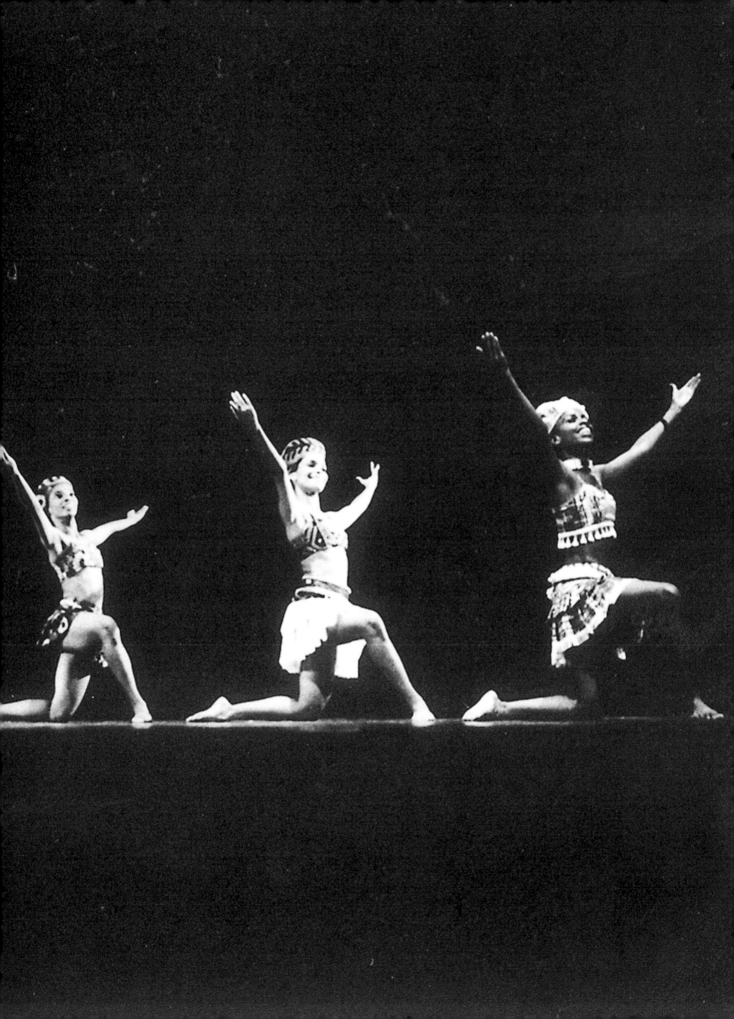

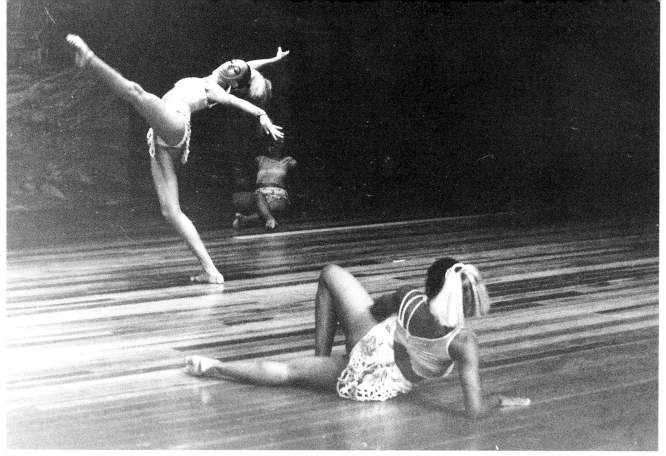

L'Acadco, 1993 Dance: Satta Choreographer: L'Antoinette Stines Dancers: N'gelle Gage & Glenda Joseph-Dennis

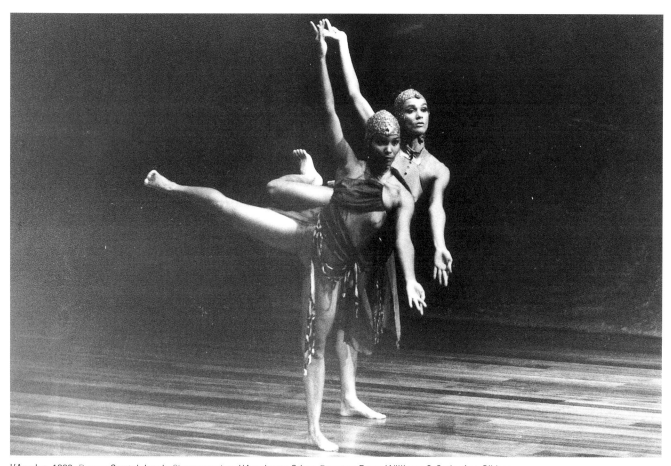

L'Acadco, 1993 Dance: Crystal Jungle Choreographer: L'Antoinette Stines Dancers: Rema Williams & Cathy Ann Gibbon

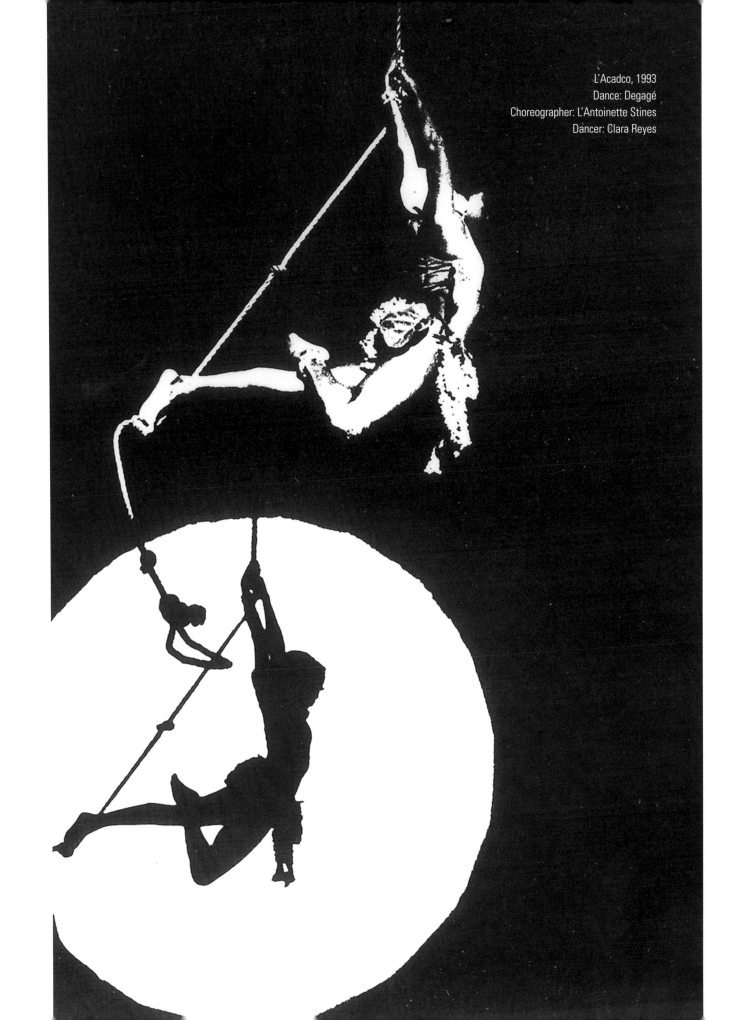

L'Acadco, 1993
Dance: Degagé
Choreographer: L'Antoinette Stines
Dancer: Clara Reyes

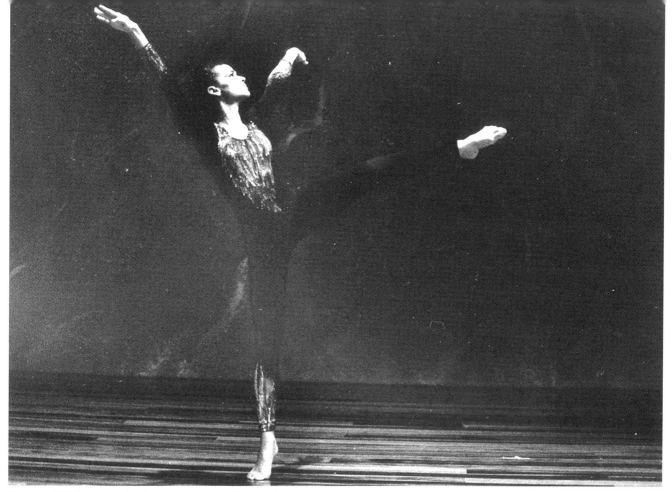

L'Acadco, 1993 Dance: The Mating Choreographer: Milton Sterling Dancer: Cathy Ann Gibbon

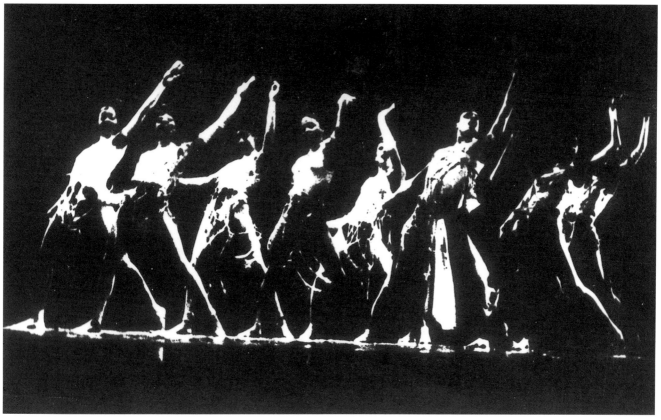

L'Acadco, 1999 Dance: Hounfour of the Drum Choreographer: L'Antoinette Stines Dancers: The Company

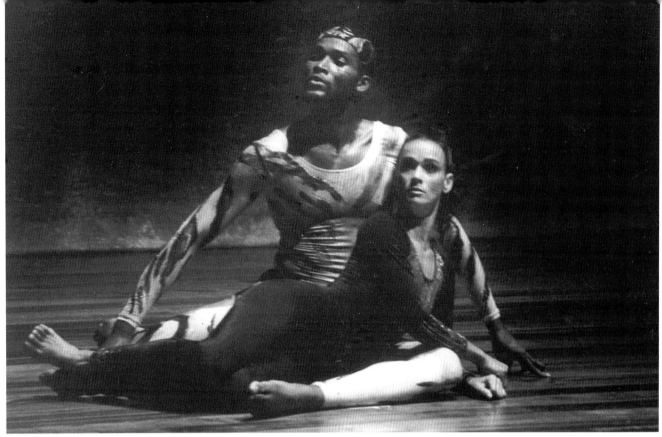

L'Acadco, 1993 Dance: The Mating Choreographer: Milton Sterling Dancers: David Browne & Cathy Ann Gibbon

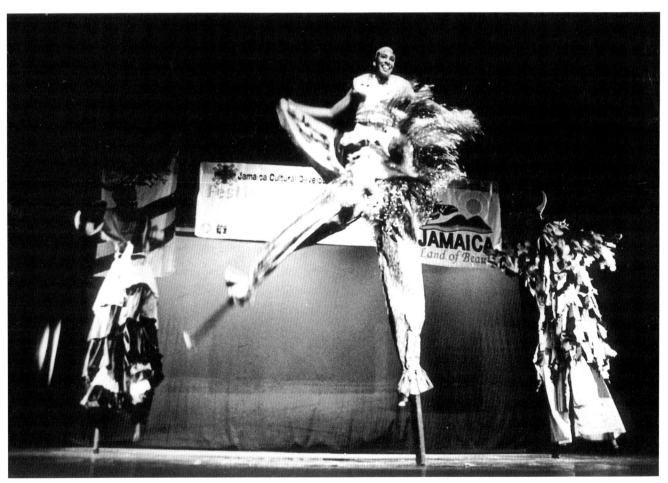

L'Acadco, 1999 Dance: Elevation Choreographer: L'Antoinette Stines Dancers: Aaron Vereen, Kafi Jones & Heron Dyce

The Company Dance Theatre

The Company Dance Theatre

The Company Dance Theatre is a product of a lifelong dream. In 1988, Tony Wilson formed the core that would become The Company Dance Theatre, and it was launched in 1989 at the Little Theatre. Since then the company has delighted and excited Jamaican audiences with its choreographic originality and energy.

The Company Dance Theatre is comprised of full company members, junior members and new recruits. Dancers who have excelled in the Junior Department are invited to take classes and learn the company repertoire. Promising dancers move from this level to junior members of the company. Tony Wilson is a dynamic teacher with innovative ideas and the gift of being able to impart them. His strong love and appreciation of music form a strong base for his works. His sense of theatre is apparent in his staging, costume and set designs for the company.

The company is a non-profit organisation run by a management committee, comprised of interested friends and supporters. All funding is provided by sponsorship from the private sector, and through donations of cash, fundraising events organised by the management committee and the company's productions.

The Company Dance Theatre has developed a distinctive repertoire of unique style and artistic creativity borne out by critical acclaim and enduring and growing audiences. It has set and maintained a reputation for a high standard of form and clarity and has displayed an abundance of vitality, high levels of training and versatility in varied and exciting programmes.

'Jamaica is a rich and multicultured country and I feel dance should be exposed to and represent all these experiences. To my mind, for the past several years, dance teaching has been limited to the style developed by the Jamaican National Dance Theatre, and not enough emphasis placed on other techniques such as ballet, Graham, etc.'

Tony Wilson, Artistic Director

… and the music that urged us

was heard from all the world

as we danced to

the songs of our own singers

and players of instruments

we made or borrowed

drawing on ancestral memory

echoing ancient themes and lore

dancing our story and our hope

for still we hear

the strings and horns

drums of Kumina, bruckins burru

and the masked dance of John Canoe

mento and quadrille, Fan, Ribbon and Hossay

for we are all this and more

mixed in our bodies

as in our minds

and in our spirit…

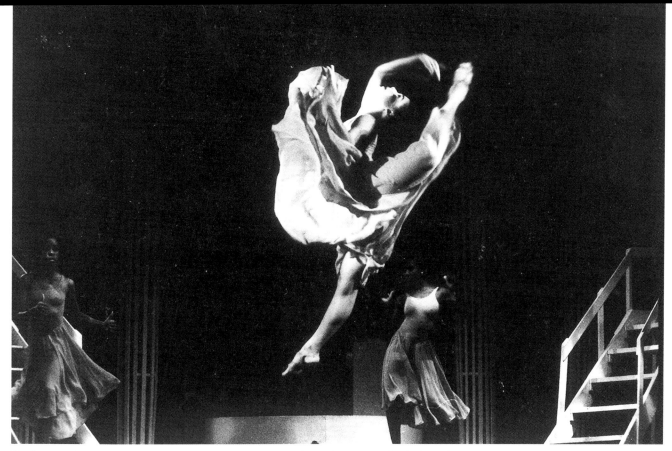

The Company Dance Theatre, 1992 Dance: Red City Choreographer: Tony Wilson Dancer: Nicola Bernard

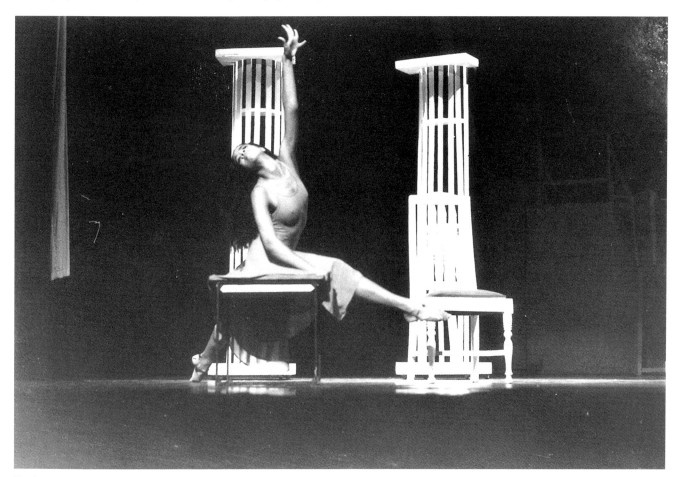

The Company Dance Theatre, 1992 Dance: Red City Choreographer: Tony Wilson Dancer: Jameela Kassim

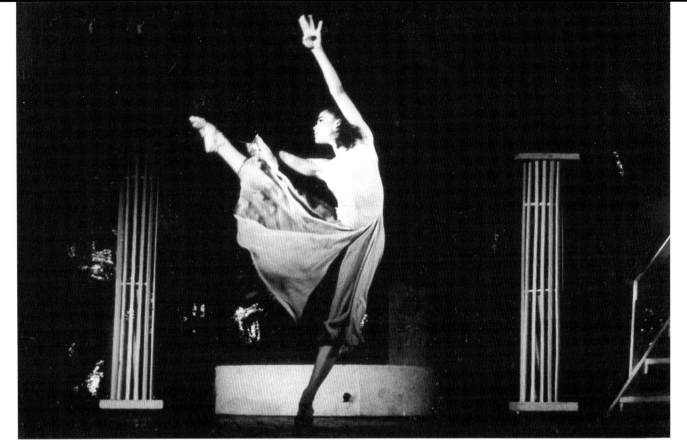

The Company Dance Theatre, 1992 Dance: Red City Choreographer: Tony Wilson Dancer: Nicola Bernard

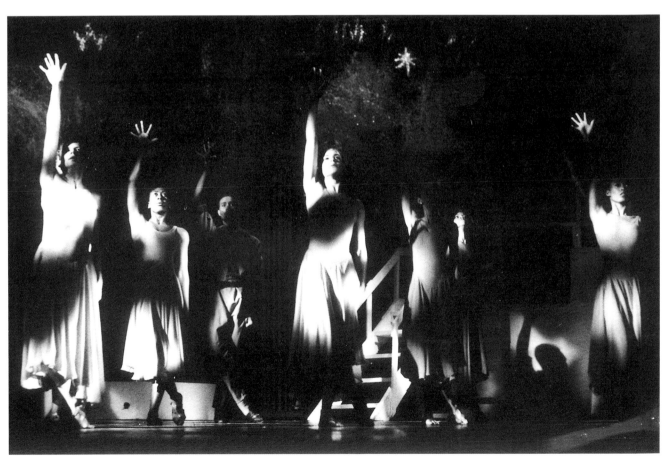

The Company Dance Theatre, 1992 Dance: Red City Choreographer: Tony Wilson Dancers: Stephanie Morecroft, Barbara McDaniel, Tony Henry, Nicola Bernard & Michelle Ward

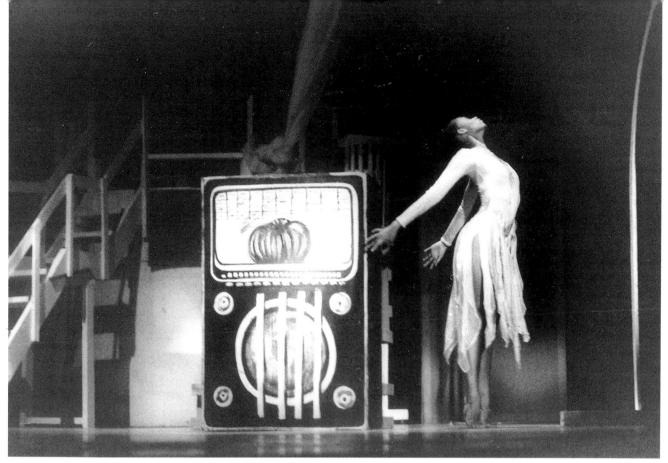

The Company Dance Theatre, 1992 Dance: Red City Choreographer: Tony Wilson Dancer: Michelle Ward

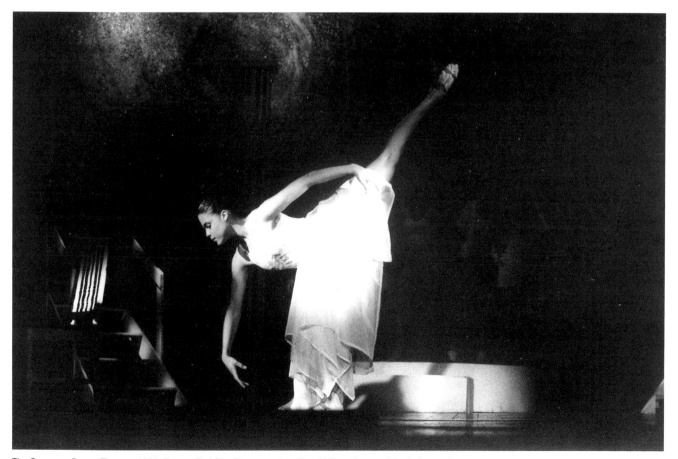

The Company Dance Theatre, 1992 Dance: Red City Choreographer: Tony Wilson Dancer: Nicola Bernard

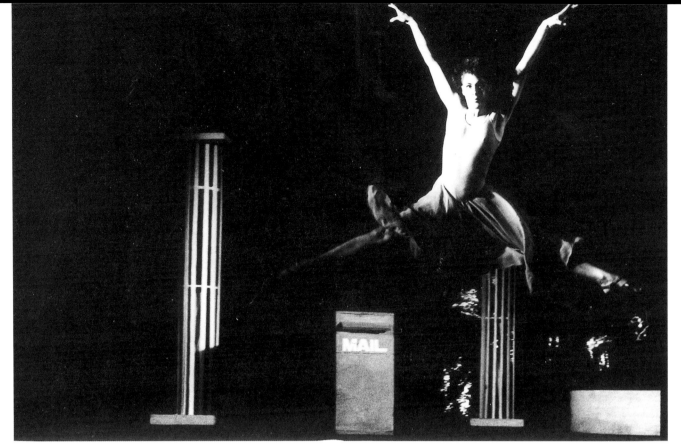

The Company Dance Theatre, 1992 Dance: Red City Choreographer: Tony Wilson Dancer: Nicola Bernard

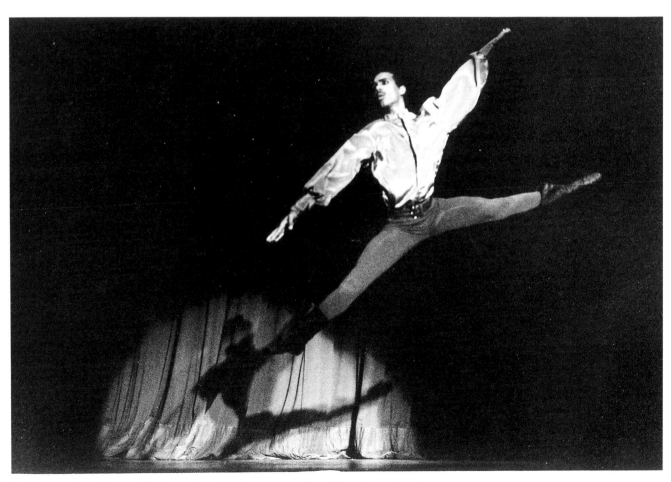

The Company Dance Theatre, 1993 Dance: Rose Hall Choreographer: Tony Wilson Dancer: Tony Henry

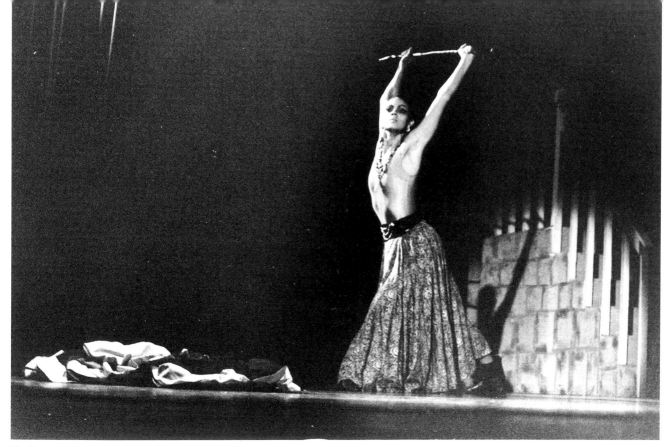

The Company Dance Theatre, 1993 Dance: Rose Hall Choreographer: Tony Wilson Dancer: Debbie Whittingham-Kerr

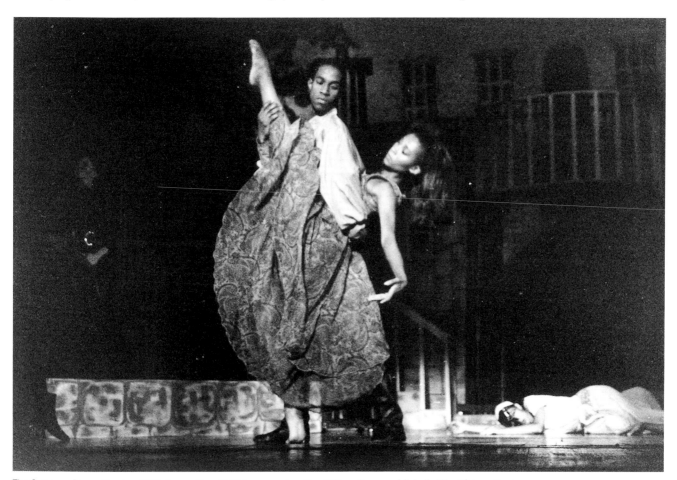

The Company Dance Theatre, 1993 Dance: Rose Hall Choreographer: Tony Wilson Dancers: Michelle Ward & Iyun Harrison

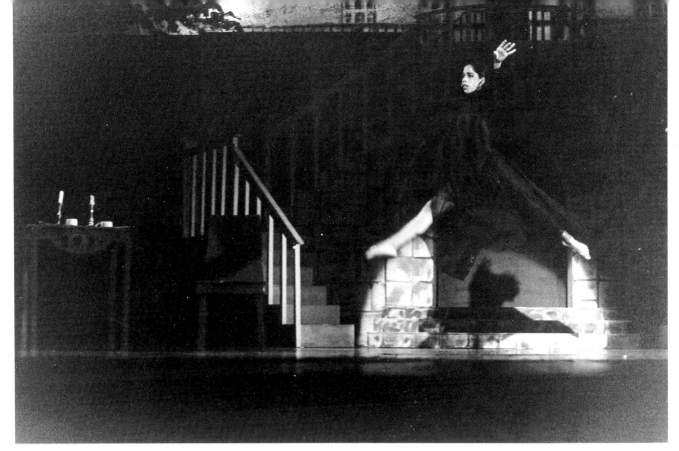

The Company Dance Theatre, 1993 Dance: Rose Hall Choreographer: Tony Wilson Dancer: Jameela Kassim

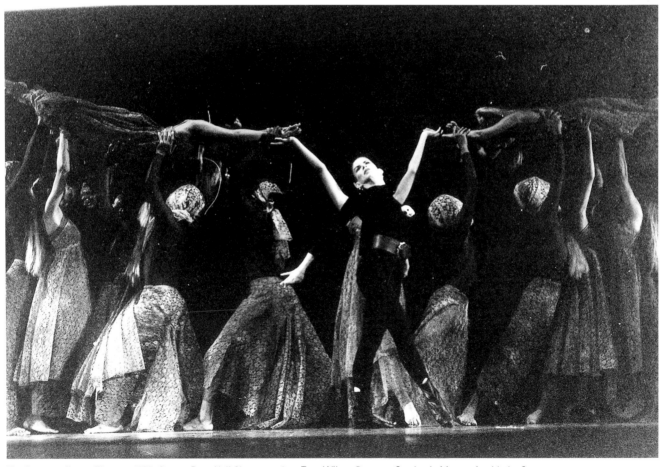

The Company Dance Theatre, 1993 Dance: Rose Hall Choreographer: Tony Wilson Dancers: Stephanie Morecroft with the Company

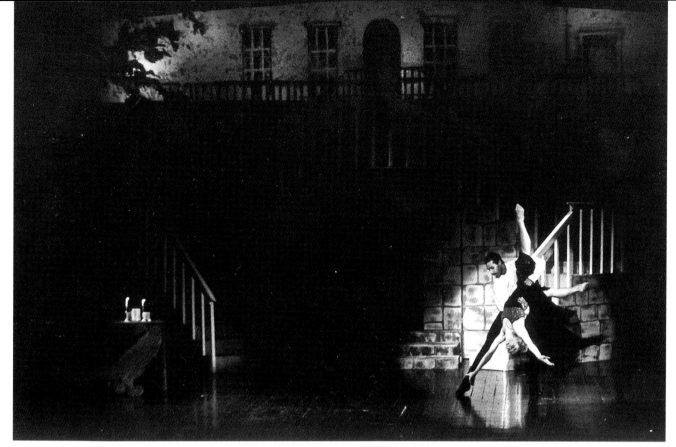

The Company Dance Theatre, 1993 Dance: Rose Hall Choreographer: Tony Wilson Dancers: Tony Henry & Stephanie Morecroft

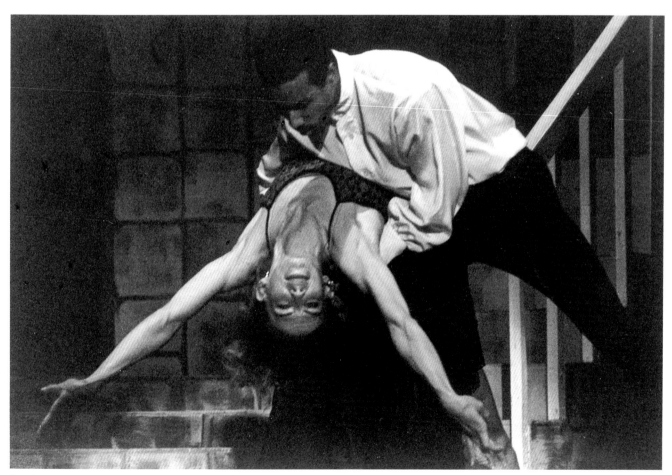

The Company Dance Theatre, 1993 Dance: Rose Hall Choreographer: Tony Wilson Dancers: Stephanie Morecroft & Tony Henry

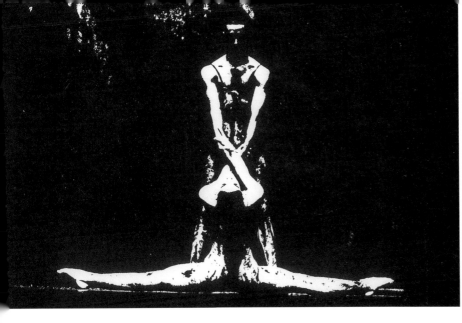

The Company Dance Theatre, 1993
Dance: Concensus
Choreographer: Tony Wilson
Dancers: Nicola Bernard & Tony Henry (Ward Theatre)

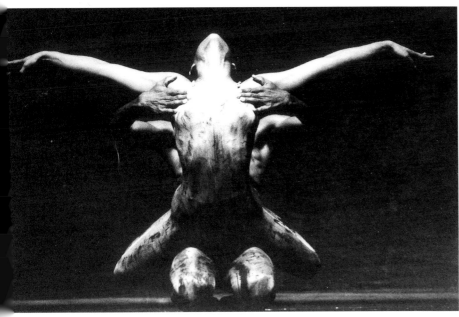

The Company Dance Theatre, 1993
Dance: Concensus
Choreographer: Tony Wilson
Dancers: Nicola Bernard & Tony Henry (Ward Theatre)

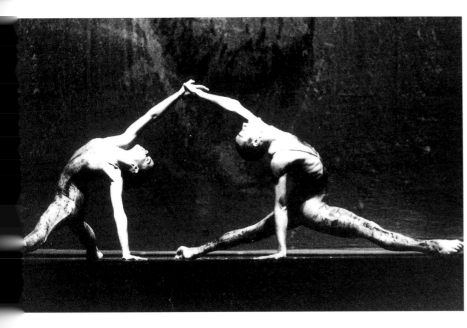

The Company Dance Theatre, 1993
Dance: Concensus
Choreographer: Tony Wilson
Dancers: Nicola Bernard & Tony Henry (Ward Theatre)

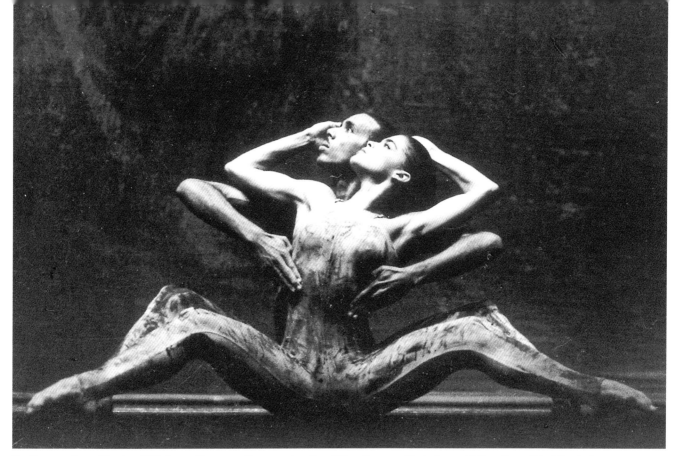

The Company Dance Theatre, 1993 Dance: Concensus Choreographer: Tony Wilson Dancers: Nicola Bernard & Tony Henry (Ward Theatre)

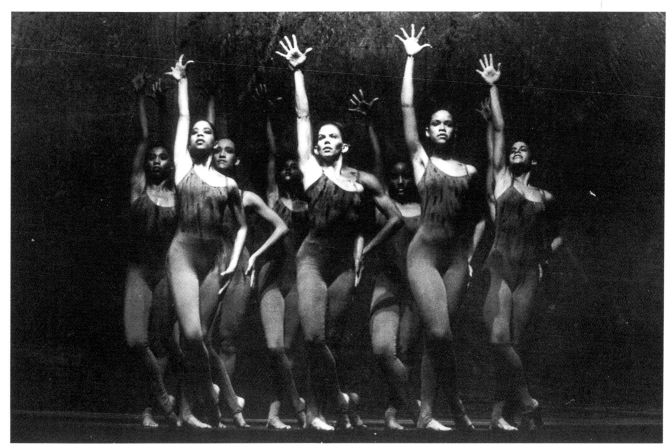

The Company Dance Theatre, 1993 Dance: Concensus Choreographer: Tony Wilson Dancers: Michelle Ward, Jameela Kassim, Lisa McLean, Trixie Macmillan, Stephanie Morecroft, Dana Lawson, Natalie Gallimore & Nicola Bernard

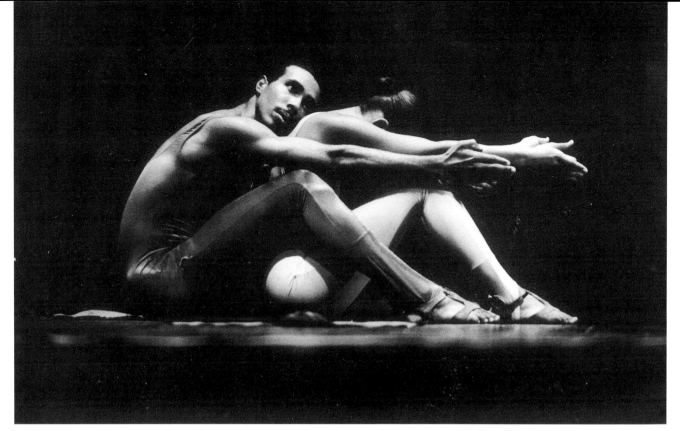

The Company Dance Theatre, 1994 Dance: Colours Choreographer: Tony Wilson Dancers: Tony Henry & Trixie Macmillan

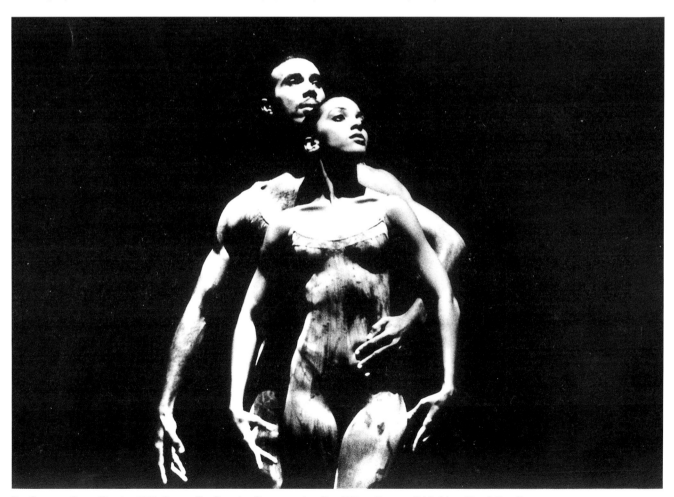

The Company Dance Theatre, 1994 Dance: The Dawning Choreographer: Tony Wilson Dancers: Trixie Macmillan & Tony Henry

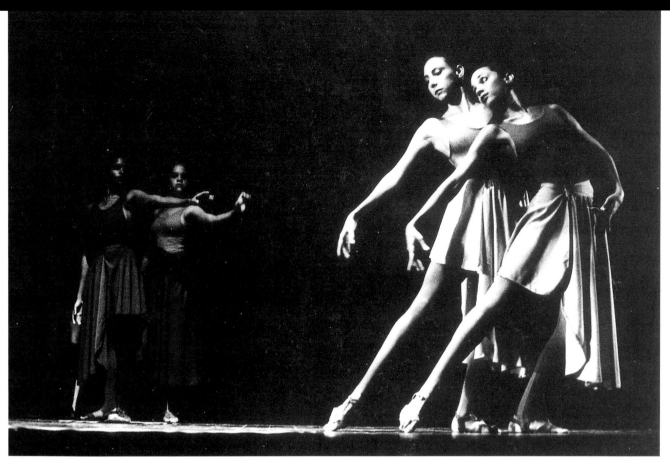

The Company Dance Theatre, 1994 Dance: Colours Choreographer: Tony Wilson Dancers: Tracy Williams & Trixie Macmillan (background Lee-Ann Steele & Kris-Ann Steele)

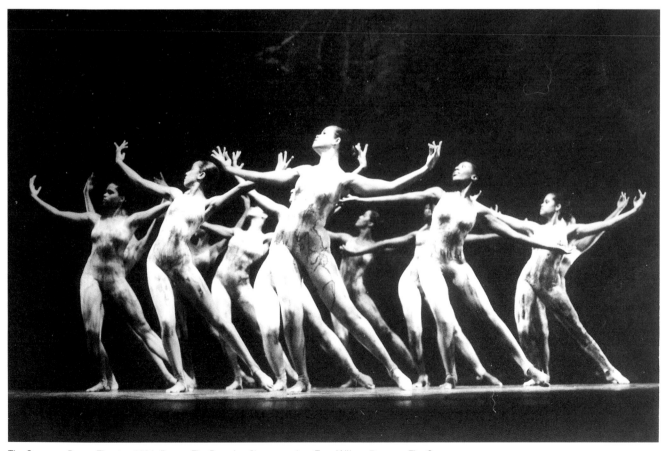

The Company Dance Theatre, 1994 Dance: The Dawning Choreographer: Tony Wilson Dancers: The Company

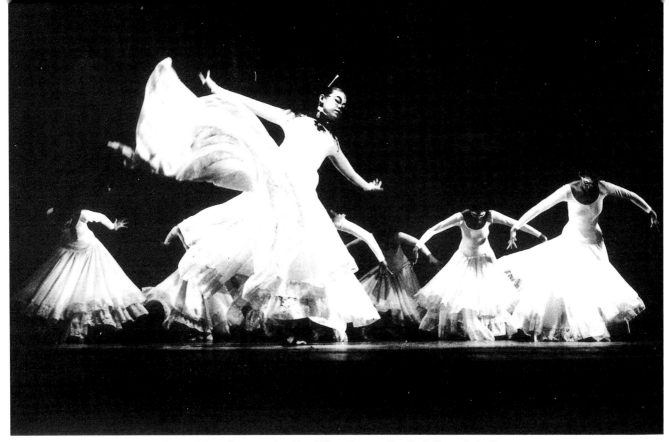

The Company Dance Theatre, 1994 Dance: Prisms Choreographer: Tony Wilson Dancers: Natalie Gallimore & the Company

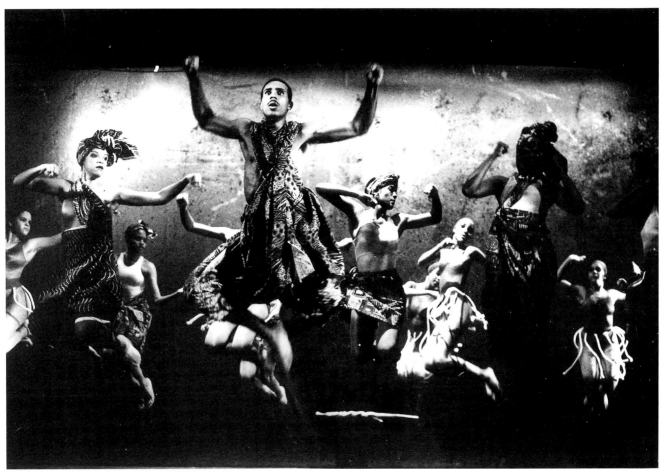

The Company Dance Theatre, 1994 Dance: Tribes Choreographer: Barbara McDaniel Dancers: The Company

The Stella Maris Dance Ensemble

The Stella Maris (Young Adult) Dance Ensemble

In 1984, a fledgling dance troupe at Stella Maris Preparatory School on Shortwood Road began an exploration of movement, under the guidance of the school's Principal, Sr Mary Josephs, and artistic director, MoniKa Lawrence. From these beginnings grew a top dance workshop which included past students (aged between 15 and 23 years) of Stella Maris Preparatory School and of other schools. In 1994, the troupe celebrated its incredible growth and considerable reputation with the launch of The Stella Maris Dance Ensemble, peopled by the senior dancers within the troupe. Since the ensemble's 1997 Season, the troupe has undergone several important changes – the most notable being an addition to its name which now sees the group being called The Stella Maris (Young Adult) Dance Ensemble. Their ballet mistress and tutor is Patsy Ricketts, and their resident tutor and choreographer is Abledo (Tokie) Gonzales Fonseca.

The Stella Maris (Young Adult) Dance Ensemble continues the long tradition of excellence in dance which was set by the Stella Maris dancers. MoniKa Lawrence is the artistic director and choreographer. Each year they have impressed judges and audiences at the Jamaica Cultural Development Commission's (JCDC) Festival Dance Competition. The company over the years has been awarded some 81 gold medals, 10 silver and 5 bronze medals for their achievement in dance. In 1989, they became the first group ever to win both the Junior and the Intermediate categories. Their consistent high achievement in the National Dance Competition also resulted in them being awarded gold medals for all 11 dances entered in 1993. After a break of three years, the senior group/ensemble re-entered the JCDC Festival Dance Competition in 1997 and, in addition to winning several gold medals for individual dances, the troupe topped the competition by winning the Ivy Baxter Trophy for the 'Best Overall Group'. They won that trophy again in 1998, to take a second consecutive – and third overall – hold on the trophy.

The dancers have also established a fine reputation overseas. In 1986, they became the youngest group to represent Jamaica overseas when they toured the Cayman Islands with 'Stella's Tale' – a Christmas pantomime produced by the school. In July 1994, the dancers also represented Jamaica at the Fourteenth Annual Caribbean Cultural Festival of Art, which was held in Santiago de Cuba. They have represented Jamaica at festivals in Mexico and Spain. In 2002, the ensemble represented Jamaica at the augural Caribbean Music Festival that was staged in Japan, as a means of forging closer cultural and economic ties between CARICOM countries and Japan. It was the first time that a Jamaican dance company performed in Japan. During that same year, the dance troupe represented Jamaica in Japan at the Sakai World Performing Festival. They have also performed in 2004 at The Black Academy of Arts and Letters in Dallas Texas, receiving rave reviews. The Stella Maris dancers have always remained true to their motto 'Success through Hard Work', and have been dedicated in their pursuit of excellence.

MoniKa Lawrence, Artistic Director

…moves the dance

with leaders bold and strong

sometimes with borrowed stance

with thanks and pride

we recall those who set the pace

Johnson, Baxter, Thomas

Soohih, Rowe and Doran

those who caught the vision

Nettleford, Campbell and Campbell

Mock-Yen, Stines, Black, Guy

Thompson, Ricketts, Wilson

Rose, Moncrieffe, Barnett and Requa

plus a host of others

in village town and city schools

shaping moulding

moving the movement

across our fair land…

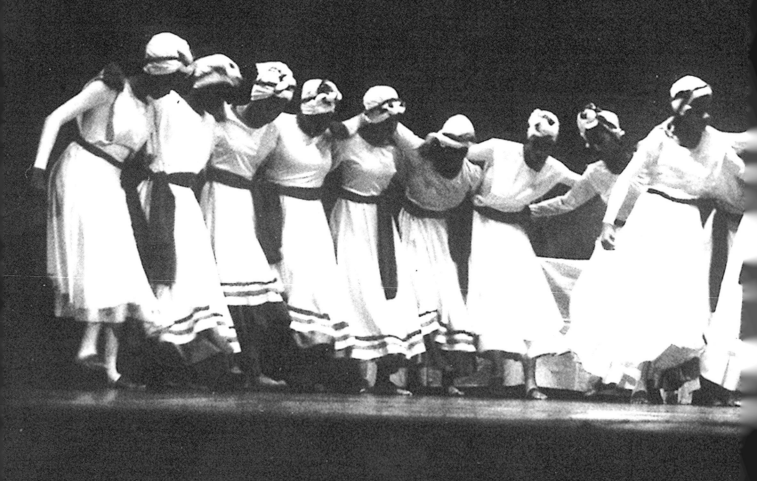

The Stella Maris Dance Ensemble, 1994
Dance: Children of Sisyphus
Choreographer: Nicoleen DeGrasse-Johnson
Dancers: The Ensemble

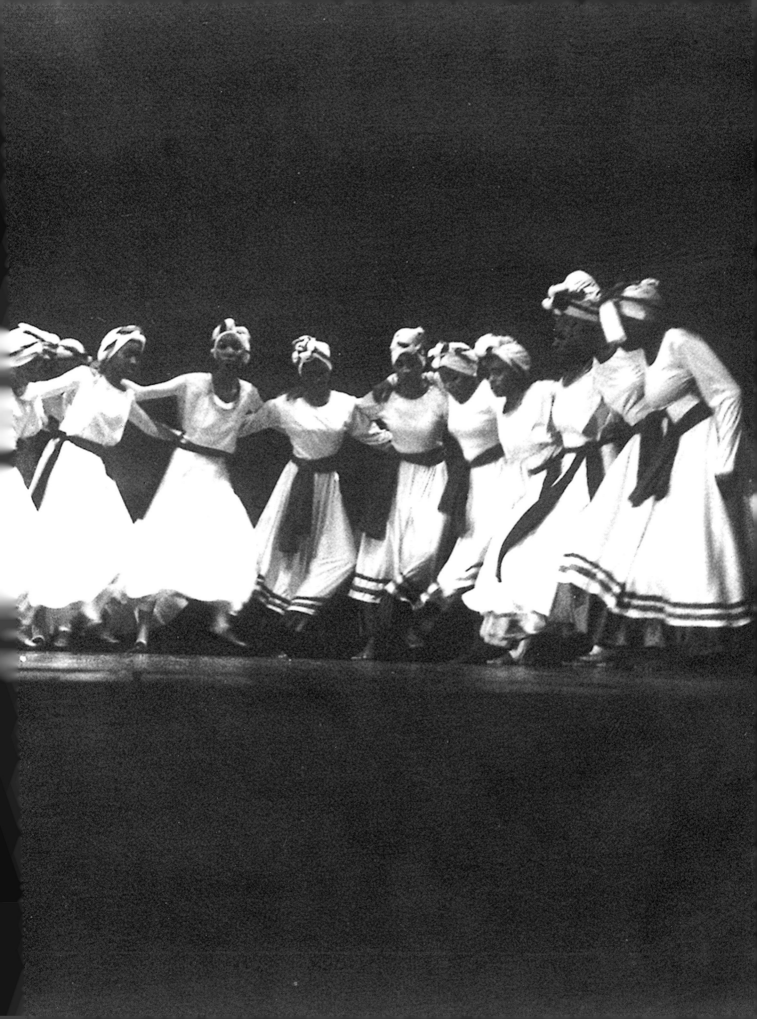

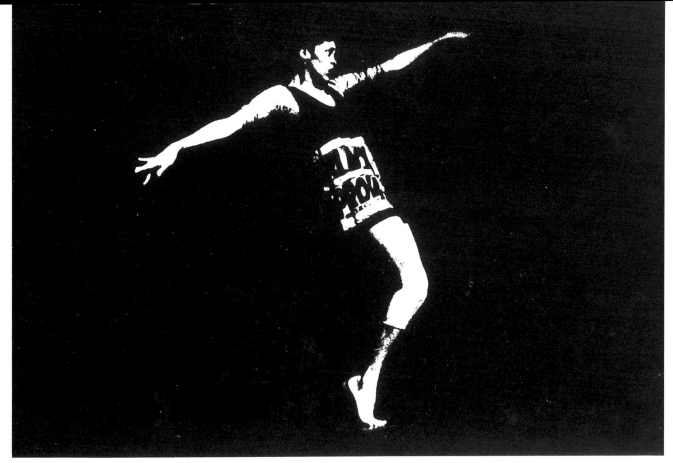

The Stella Maris Dance Ensemble, 1994   Dance: Children of Sisyphus Choreographer: MoniKa Lawrence Dancer: Neila Ebanks

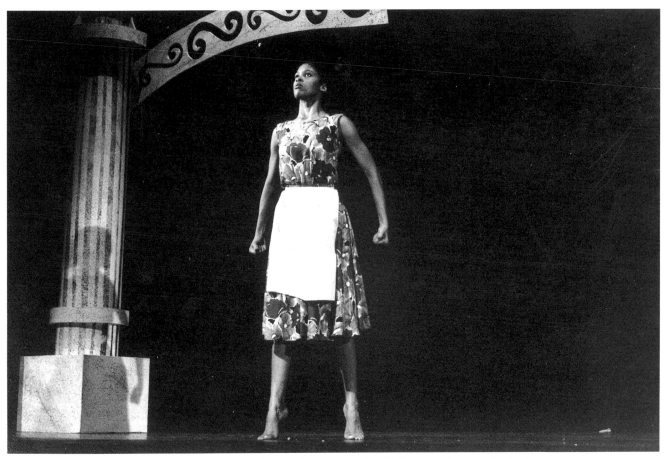

The Stella Maris Dance Ensemble, 1994   Dance: Children of Sisyphus Choreographer: MoniKa Lawrence Dancer: Neila Ebanks

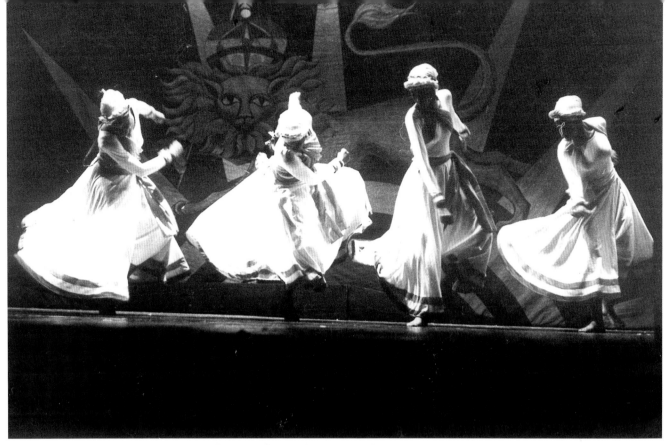

The Stella Maris Dance Ensemble, 1994 Dance: Children of Sisyphus Choreographer: MoniKa Lawrence Dancers: Patsy Ricketts & the Ensemble

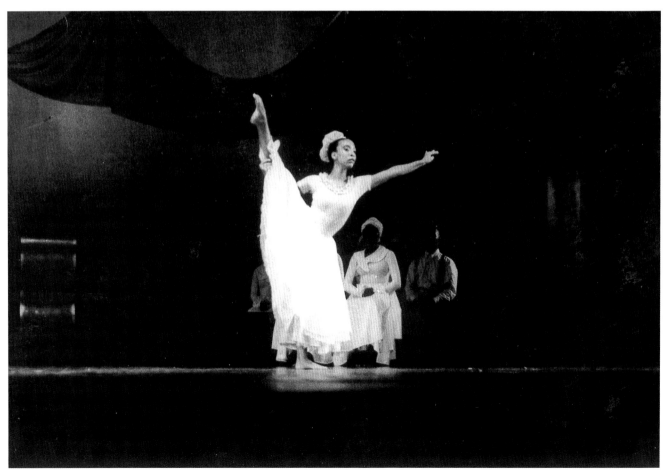

The Stella Maris Dance Ensemble, 1995 Dance: The Seventh Day Choreographer: MoniKa Lawrence Dancer: Wendi Hoofatt

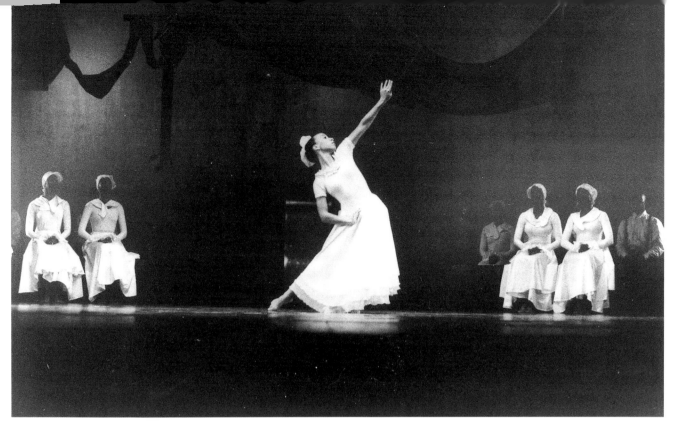

The Stella Maris Dance Ensemble, 1995 Dance: The Seventh Day Choreographer: MoniKa Lawrence Dancers: Wendi Hoofatt & the Ensemble

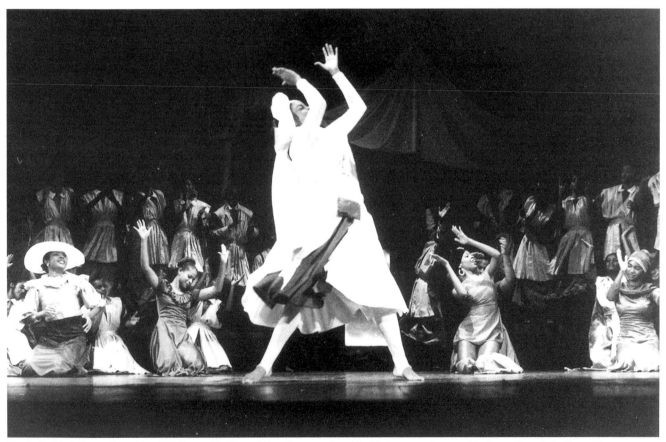

The Stella Maris Dance Ensemble, 1995 Dance: The Seventh Day Choreographer: MoniKa Lawrence Dancers: Meshagae Hunt & the Ensemble

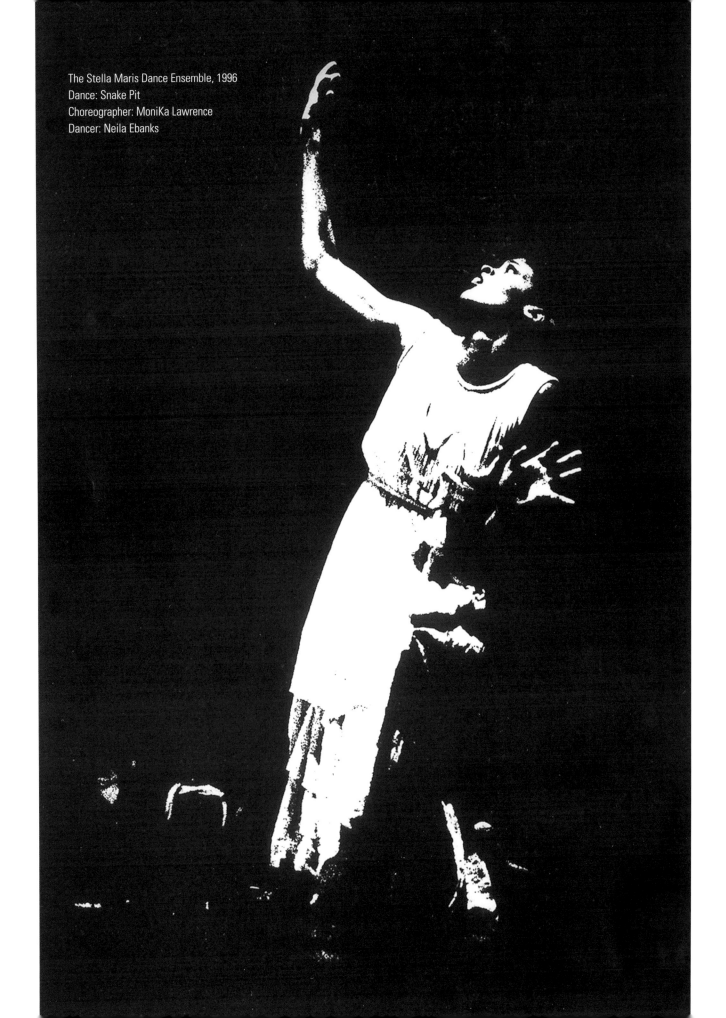

The Stella Maris Dance Ensemble, 1996
Dance: Snake Pit
Choreographer: MoniKa Lawrence
Dancer: Neila Ebanks

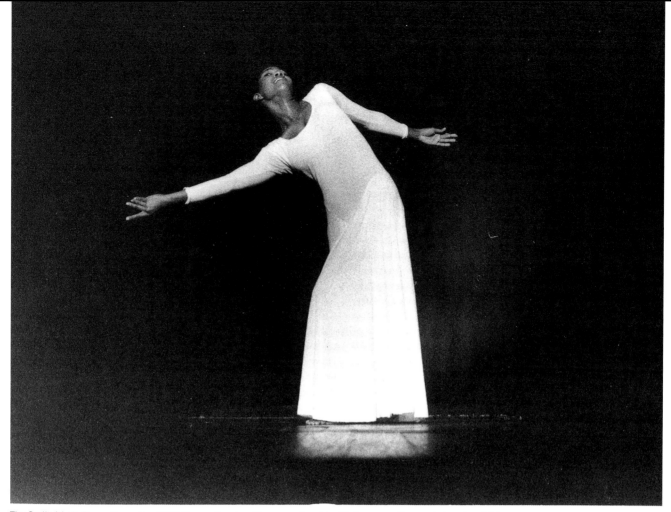

The Stella Maris Dance Ensemble, 1996 Dance: Freedom Choreographer: MoniKa Lawrence Dancer: Latoya Lyseight

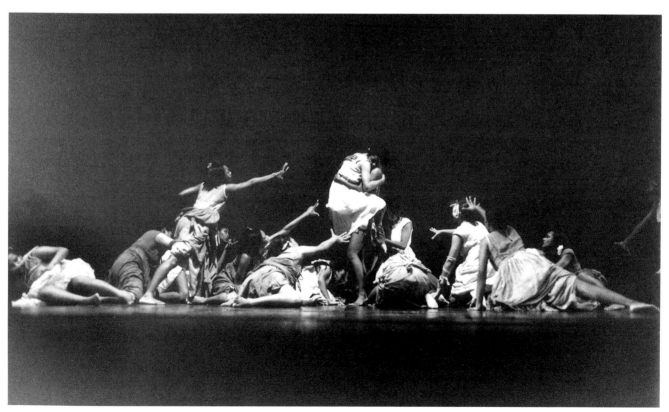

The Stella Maris Dance Ensemble, 1996 Dance: Snake Pit Choreographer: MoniKa Lawrence Dancers: The Ensemble

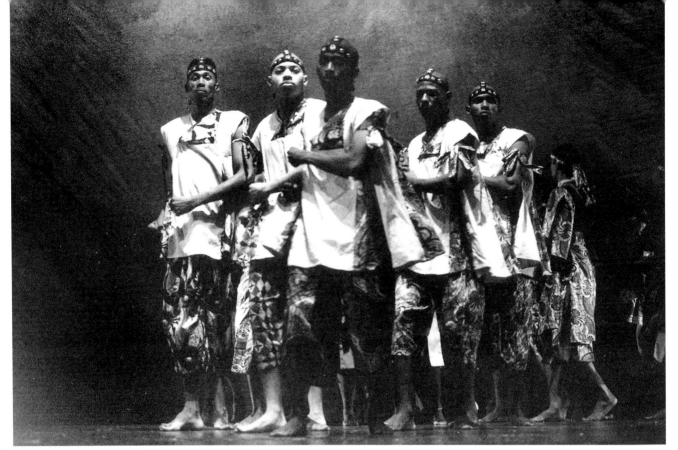

The Stella Maris Dance Ensemble, 1996 Dance: Dance Jallof Choreographer: 'H' Patten Dancers: Errol Moodie, Garth Anderson, Gregory Beckles, Mark Weir & Andrew Brown

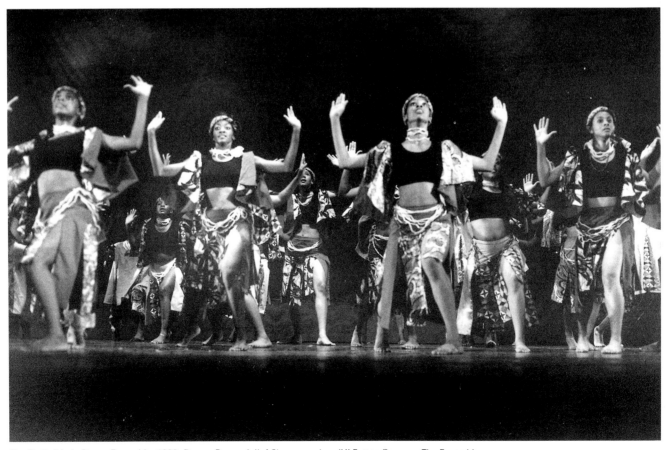

The Stella Maris Dance Ensemble, 1996 Dance: Dance Jallof Choreographer: 'H' Patten Dancers: The Ensemble

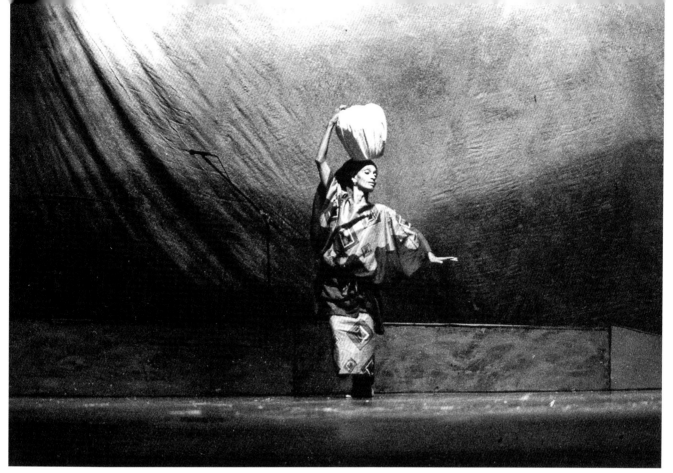

The Stella Maris Dance Ensemble, 1996 Dance: Dance Jallof Choreographer: 'H' Patten Dancer: Patsy Ricketts

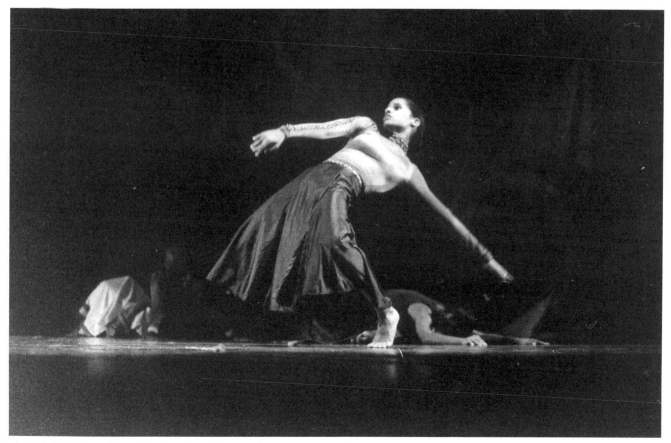

The Stella Maris Dance Ensemble, 1997 Dance: Moments Choreographer: Patsy Ricketts Dancer: Tiffany Martin

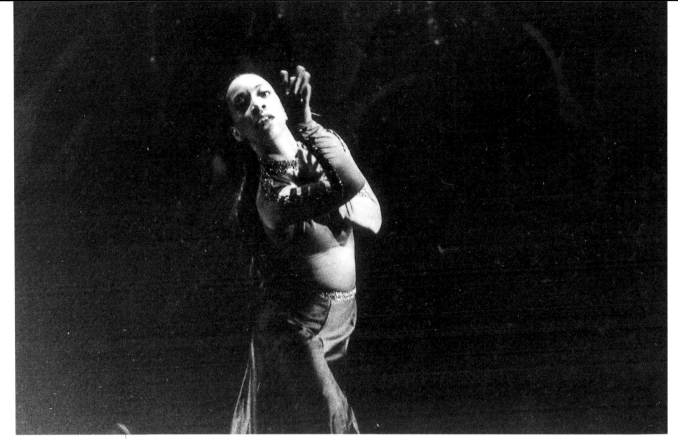

The Stella Maris Dance Ensemble, 1997 Dance: Moments Choreographer: Patsy Ricketts Dancer: Wendi Hoofatt

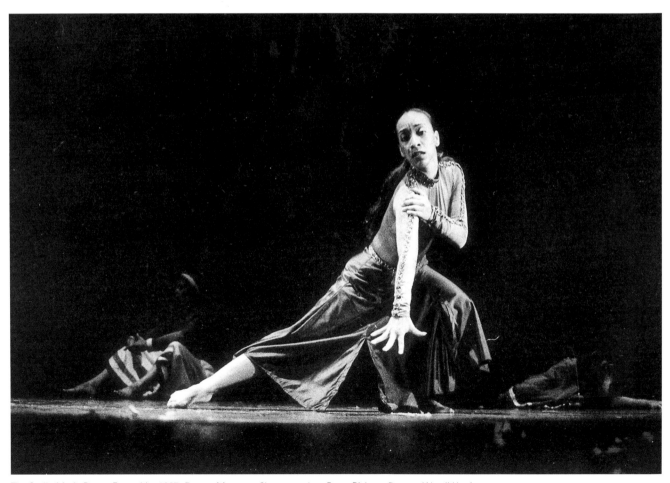

The Stella Maris Dance Ensemble, 1997 Dance: Moments Choreographer: Patsy Ricketts Dancer: Wendi Hoofatt

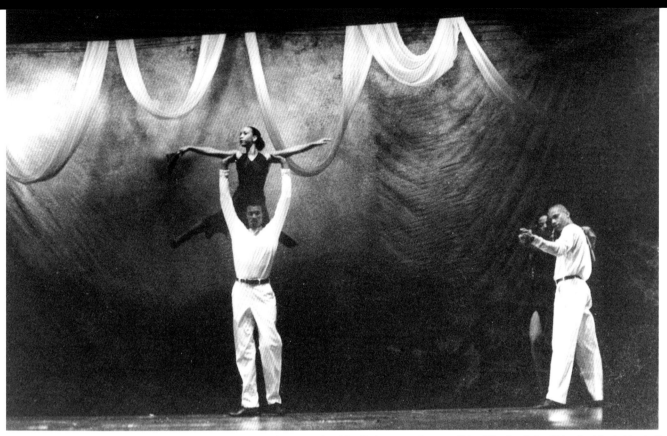

The Stella Maris Dance Ensemble, 1996   Dance: What A World Choreographer: MoniKa Lawrence Dancers: Wendi Hoofatt & Errol Moodie, Nicole Marshall & Garth Anderson

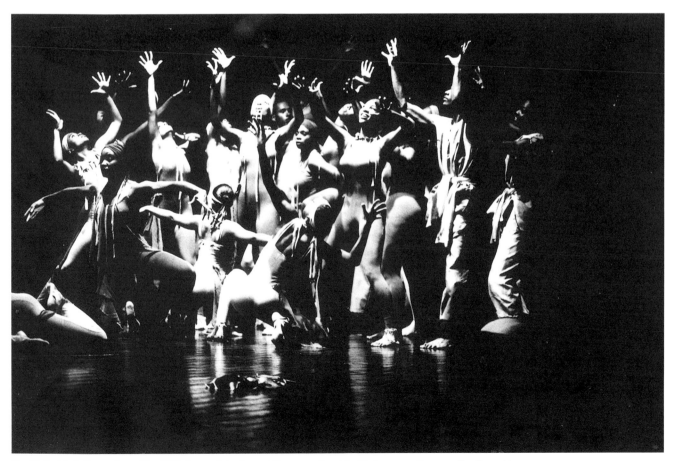

The Stella Maris Dance Ensemble, 1997   Dance: Baka Beyond Choreographer: MoniKa Lawrence Dancers: The Ensemble

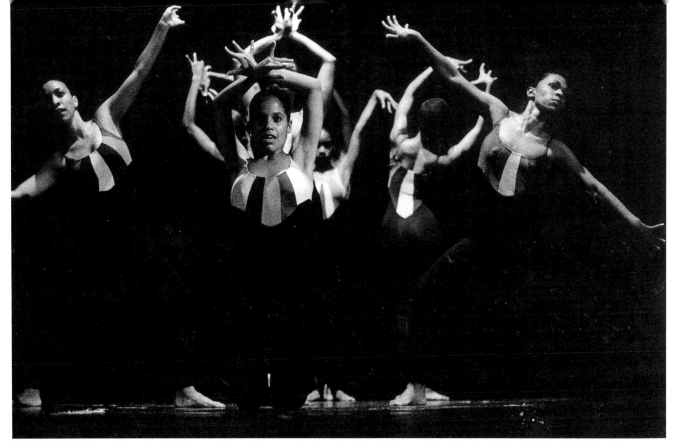

The Stella Maris Dance Ensemble, 1997 Dance: Space Choreographer: Arsenio Andrade Dancers: Wendi Hoofatt, Tiffany Martin, Keisha Singh & the Ensemble

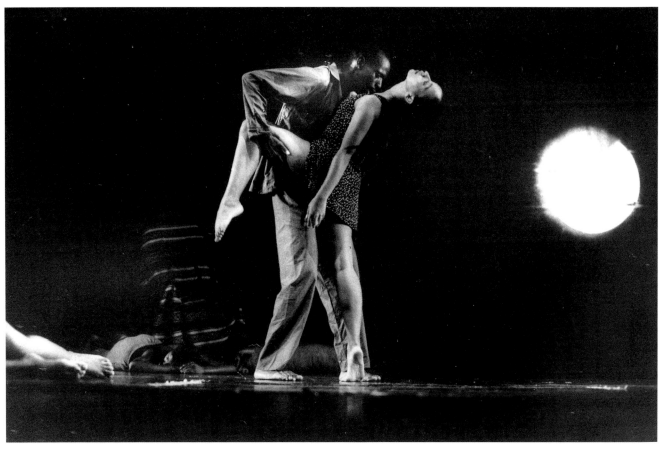

The Stella Maris Dance Ensemble, 1997 Dance: Morpheus Webb Choreographer: Nicoleen Degrasse-Johnson Dancers: Wendi Hoofatt & Ricardo Martin

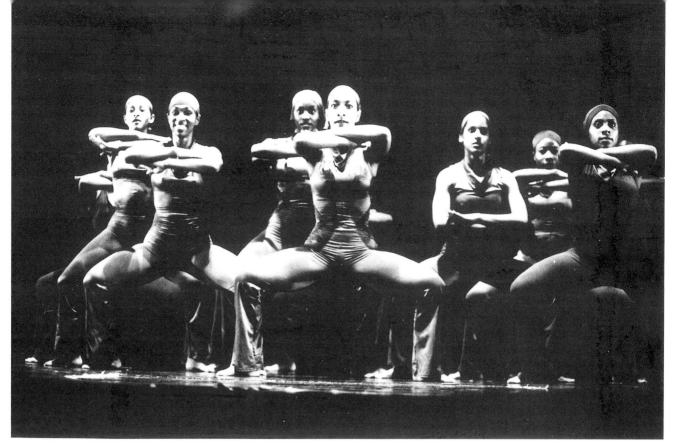

The Stella Maris Dance Ensemble, 1997 Dance: No Frills Choreographer: Neila Ebanks Dancers: Felice Mah-Leong, Keisha Singh, Karen Seymour, Wendi Hoofatt, Tiffany Martin, Marcia Lewis & Meshagae Hunt

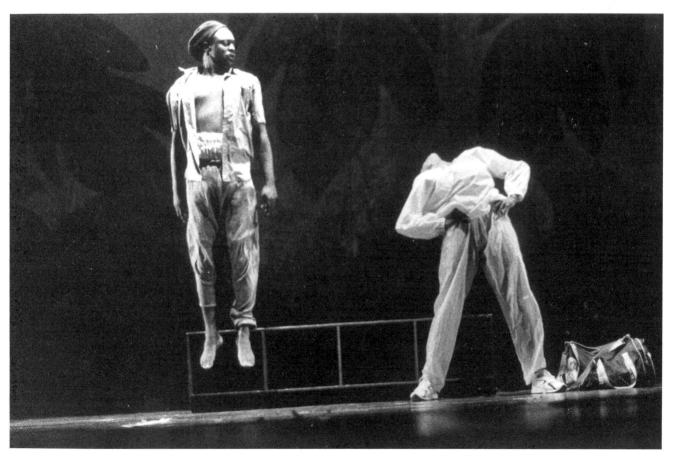

The Stella Maris Dance Ensemble, 1997 Dance: The Bench Choreographer: MoniKa Lawrence Dancers: Glen Campbell & Karen Seymour

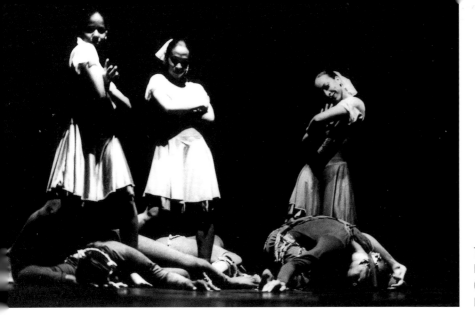

The Stella Maris Dance Ensemble, 1998
Dance: Bida Floral
Choreographer: Abeldo Gonzales
Dancers: Tiffany Martin, Keisha Singh & Wendi Hoofatt

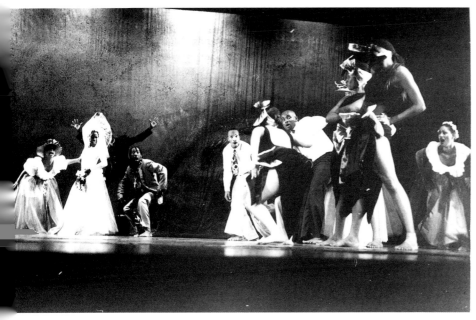

The Stella Maris Dance Ensemble, 1998
Dance: Liza
Choreographer: MoniKa Lawnence
Dancers: The Ensemble

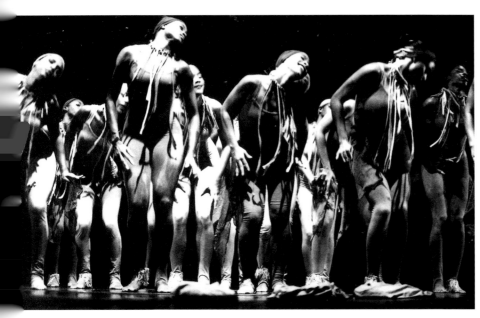

The Stella Maris Dance Ensemble, 1998
Dance: Baka Beyond
Choreographer: MoniKa Lawrence
Dancers: The Ensemble

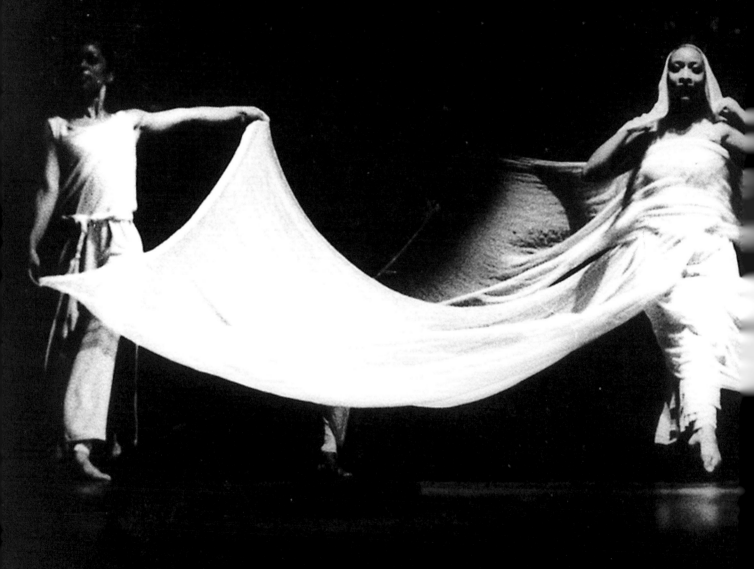

The Stella Maris Dance Ensemble, 1998
Dance: Where is Maria?
Choreographer: MoniKa Lawrence
Dancers: Tiffany Martin & Wendi Hoofatt

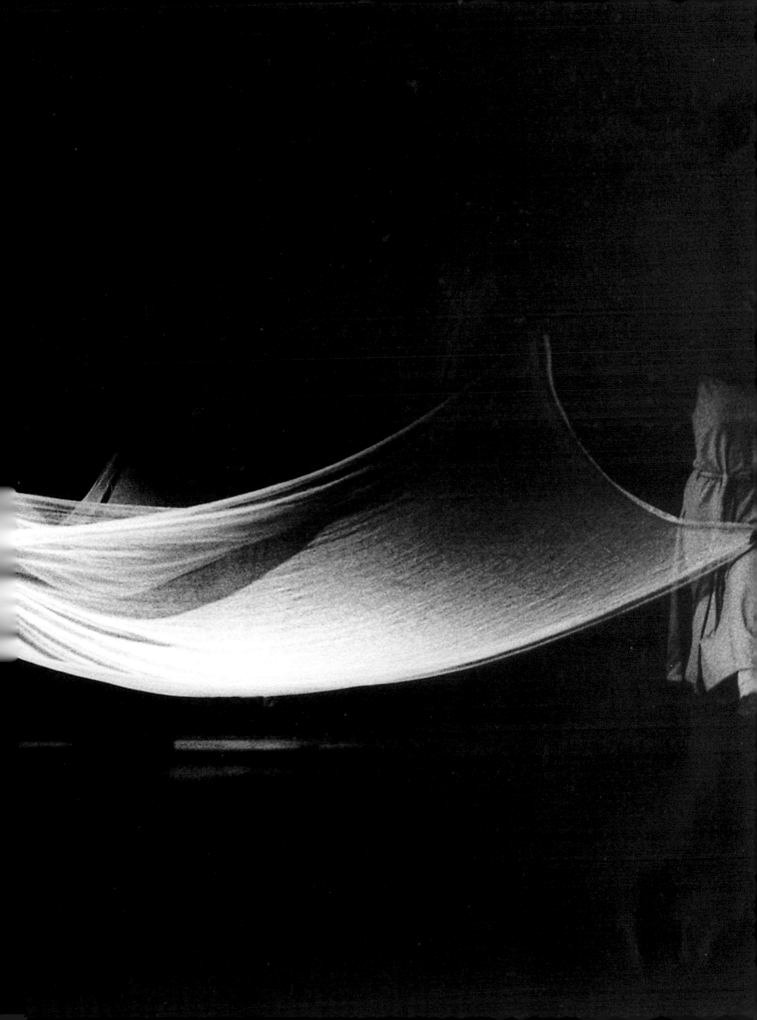

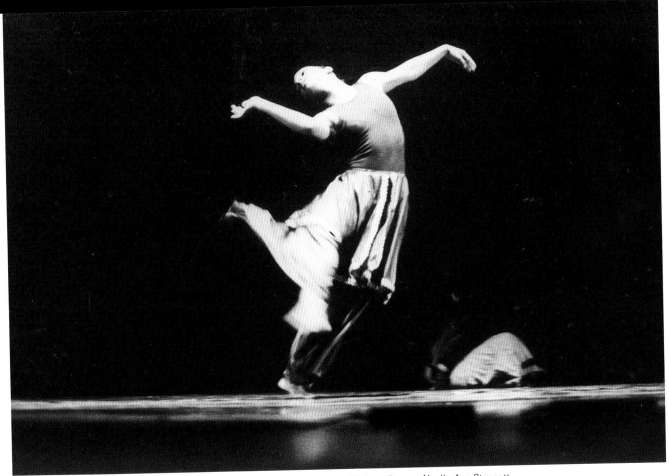

The Stella Maris Dance Ensemble, 1998 Dance: Moments Choreographer: Patsy Ricketts Dancer: Noelle-Ann Stennett

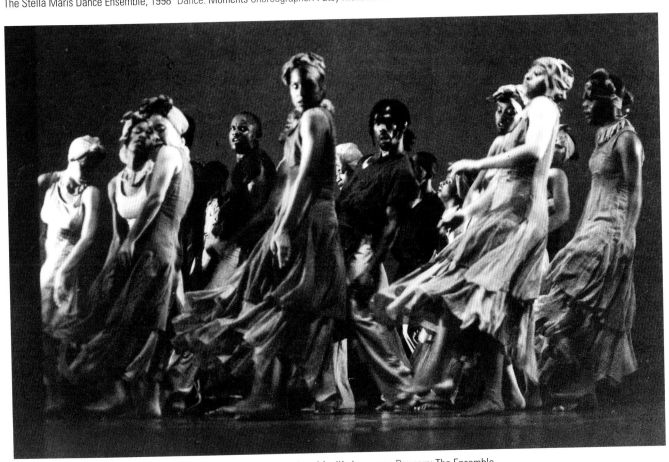

The Stella Maris Dance Ensemble, 2002 Dance: Echoes Choreographer: MoniKa Lawrence Dancers: The Ensemble

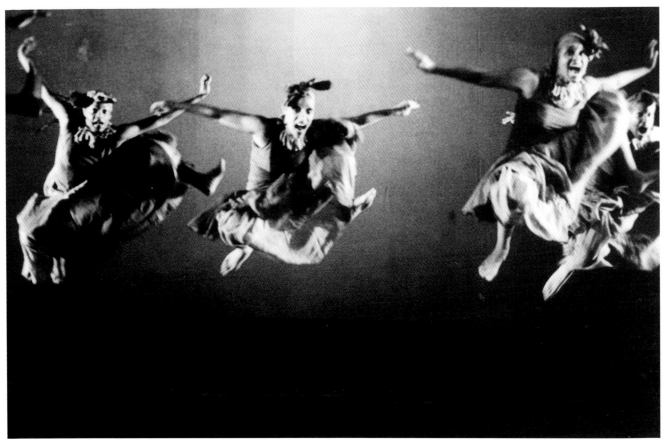

The Stella Maris Dance Ensemble, 2002 Dance: Echoes Choreographer: MoniKa Lawrence Dancers: Toni Ann Aiken, Wendi Hoofatt, Felice Mah-Leong & Tiffany Martin

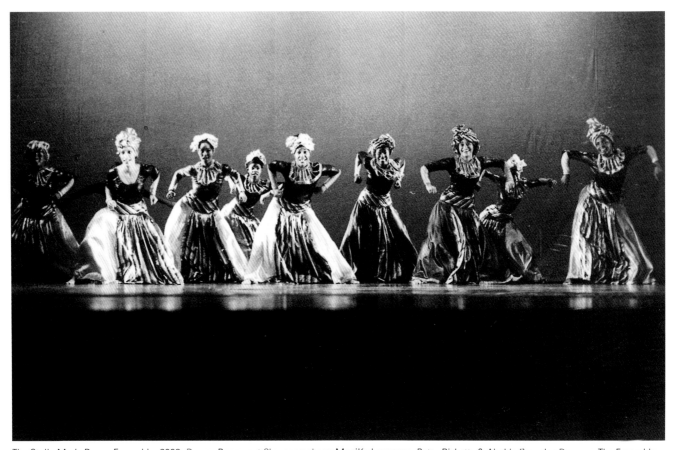

The Stella Maris Dance Ensemble, 2002 Dance: Pepperpot Choreographers: MoniKa Lawrence, Patsy Ricketts & Abeldo Gonzales Dancers: The Ensemble

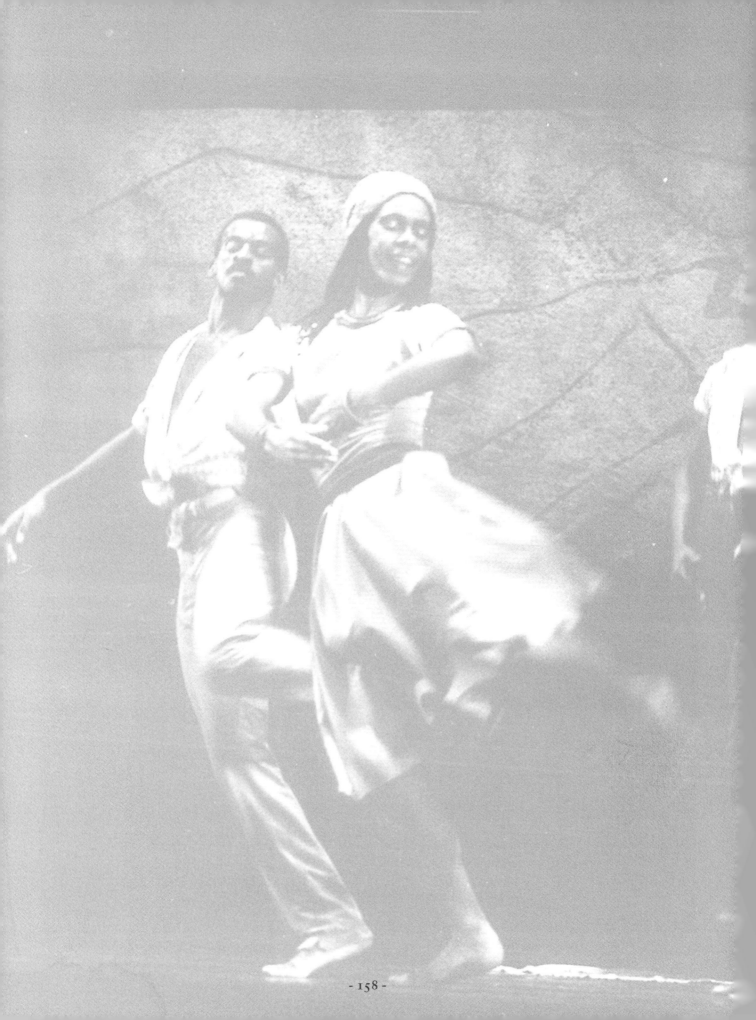

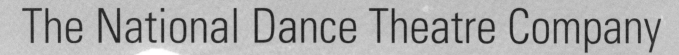

The National Dance Theatre Company

The National Dance Theatre Company

The National Dance Theatre Company of Jamaica (NDTC) was formed in 1962, at the time of Jamaica's Independence, by co-founders Rex Nettleford and Eddy Thomas (along with 16 other dedicated enthusiasts). The original 18 members represented a diverse mixture of artists, with differing backgrounds in dance training and performance from the Martha Graham School of Contemporary Dance, the Ivy Baxter Creative Dance Group, the Soohih School, the Eddy Thomas Dance Workshop, the Faye Simpson School and the Gordon Rumsey School of Dance. This emerging corps had worked together for three years in Little Theatre Movement (LTM) pantomusicals, prior to the launching of the NDTC in 1962.

The company has survived on a vision of 'dancing on its own feet', capturing the rhythms, body language, aesthetics and sense and sensibility of a people who had lived for over three centuries under British rule, and a total of 400 years under slavery and the plantation system. It has gained an international reputation, garnering both critical and audience acclaim throughout the world with its wide-ranging repertoire presented by dancers, singers, musicians and creative technicians.

To date, the NDTC has completed more than 100 tours of North America, Europe, the former USSR, Australia, the United Kingdom, Latin America, the Caribbean and Puerto Rico, and engages the Jamaican population in unbroken annual Seasons of Dance at the Little Theatre in Kingston.

Rex Nettleford, Artistic Director

…and here we proudly celebrate

the birth of our style

the movements of our dance

our dance movement growing

caught in this time and this space

as with all the disparate elements

bequeathed inherited

fused by the dancers will and spirit

we create this thing

unique special

so awesome in power and beauty

we begin to feel our presence and our worth

for that too was part of vision and purpose

and now for those to come

who will add their share

captured and frozen in time

with camera and with skill..

…and it is good.

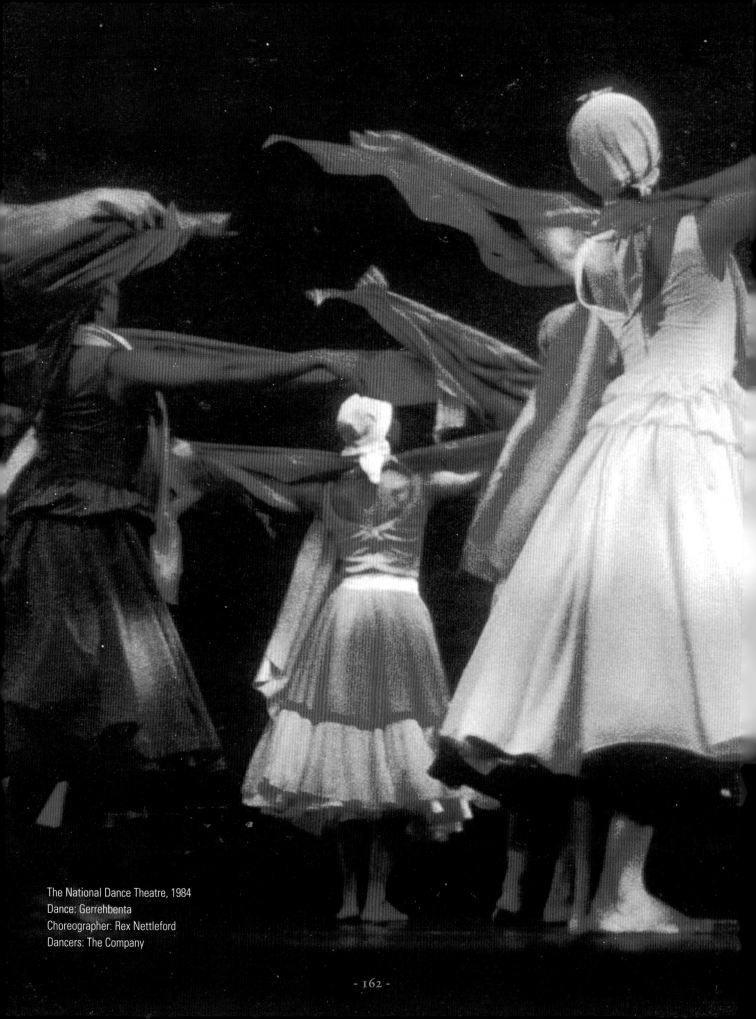

The National Dance Theatre, 1984
Dance: Gerrehbenta
Choreographer: Rex Nettleford
Dancers: The Company

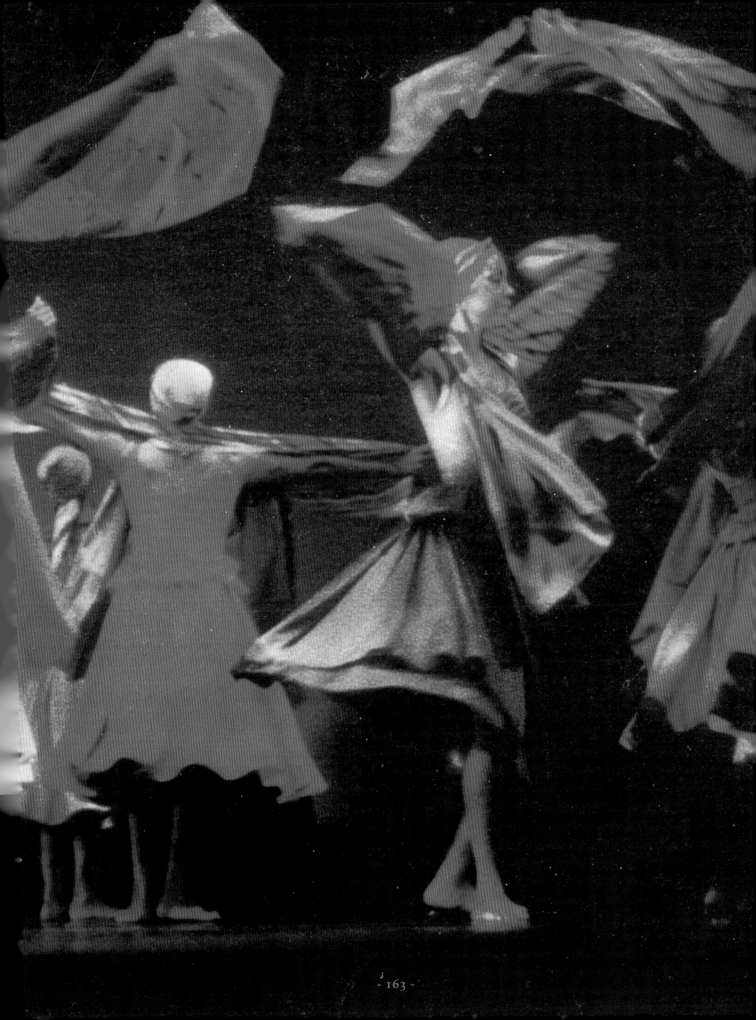

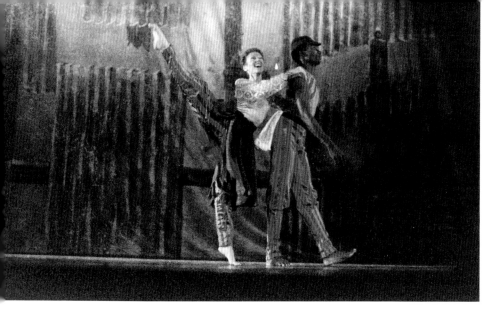

The National Dance Theatre, 1984
Dance: Vibrations
Choreographer: Rex Nettleford Dancers: Melanie
Graham & Deroi Rose

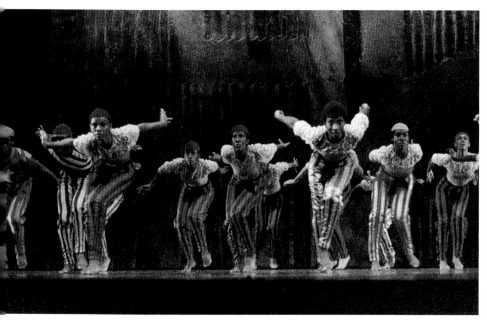

The National Dance Theatre, 1984
Dance: Vibrations
Choreographer: Rex Nettleford
Dancers: Monthy Williams, Arlene Richards,
Denise Robinson, Gabrielle Harban, Allison
Symes, Paula Monroe & MoniKa Lawrence

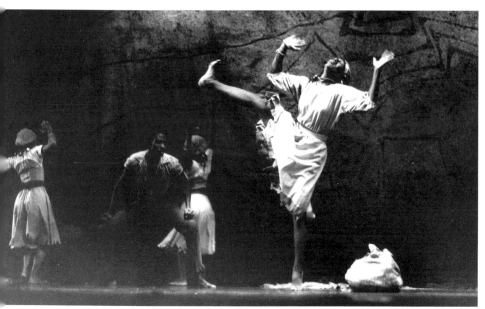

The National Dance Theatre, 1984
Dance: Dream on Squatters' Mountain
Choreographer: Rex Nettleford
Dancer: Gabrielle Harban

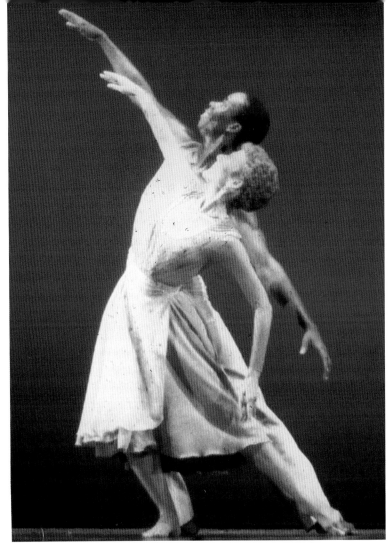

The National Dance Theatre Company, 1984
Dance: Encounters
Choreographer: Bert Rose
Dancers: Melanie Graham & Christopher Morrison

The National Dance Theatre Company, 1984
Dance: Dream on Squatters' Mountain
Choreographer: Rex Nettleford
Dancers: Eisenhower Williams & Tony Wilson

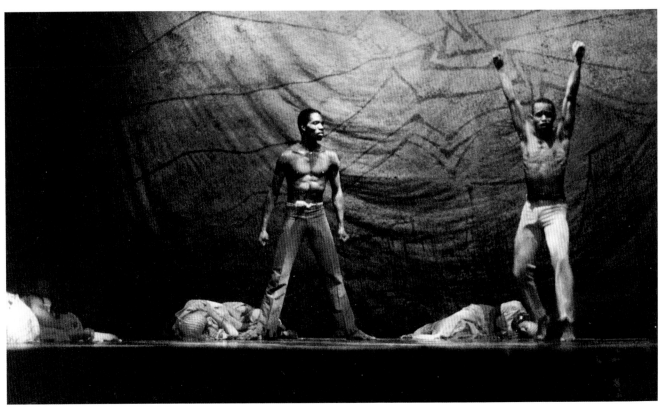

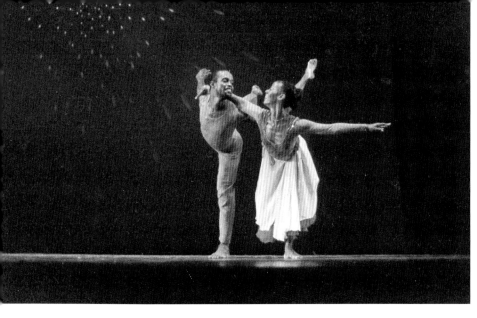

The National Dance Theatre Company, 1984
Dance: Encounters
Choreographer: Bert Rose
Dancers: Tony Wilson & MoniKa Lawrence

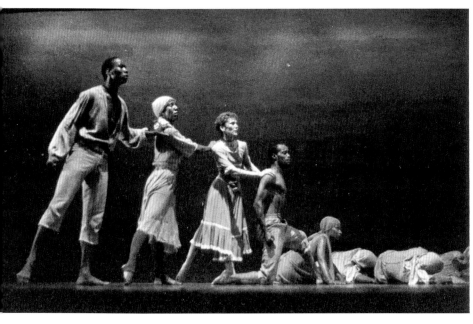

The National Dance Theatre Company, 1984
Dance: The Crossing
Choreographer: Rex Nettleford
Dancers: Christopher Morrison, Gabrielle Harban,
Melanie Graham, Tony Wilson & Judith Pennant

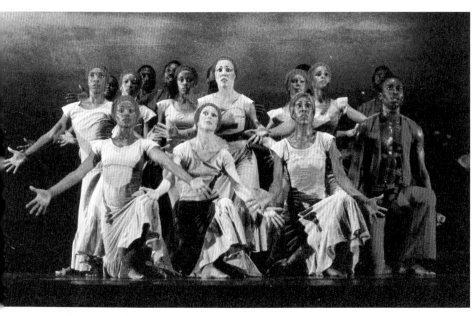

The National Dance Theatre Company, 1984
Dance: The Crossing
Choreographer: Rex Nettleford
Dancers: The Company

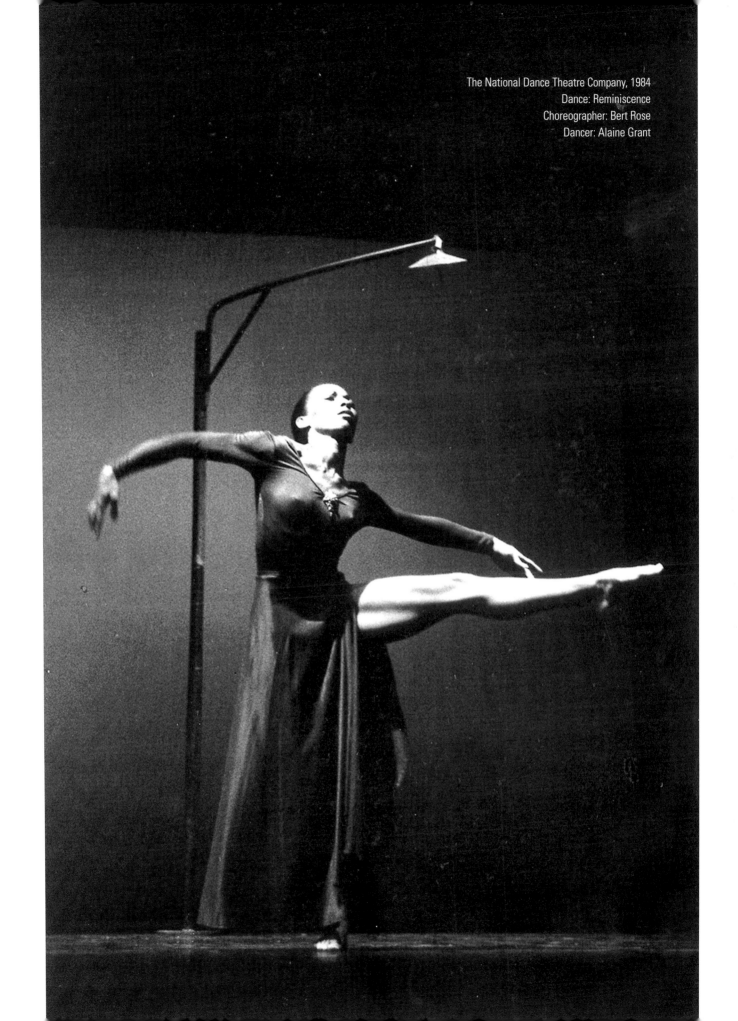

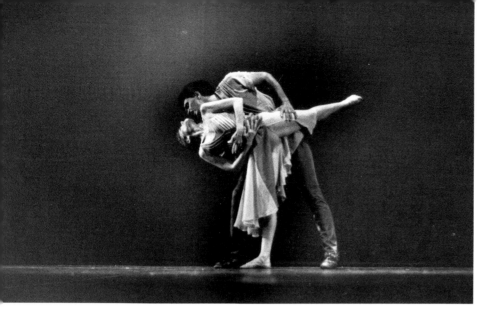

The National Dance Theatre Company, 1984
Dance: Recollections
Choreographer: Clive Thompson
Dancers: Clive Thompson & Melanie Graham

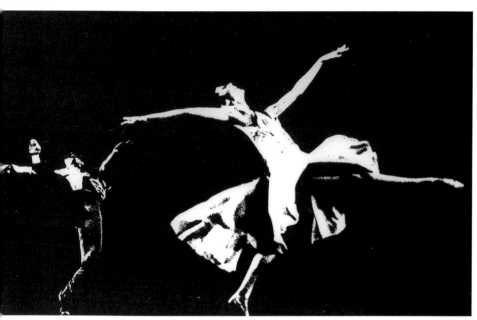

The National Dance Theatre Company, 1984
Dance: Recollections
Choreographer: Clive Thompson
Dancers: Clive Thompson & Melanie Graham

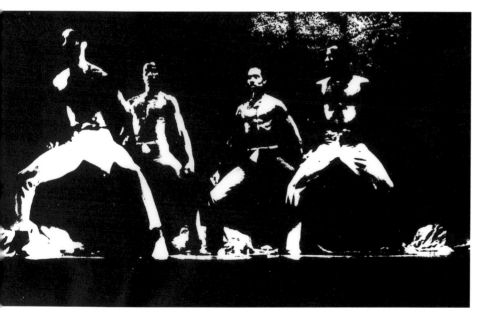

The National Dance Theatre Company, 1984
Dance: Dream on Squatters' Mountain
Choreographer: Rex Nettleford
Dancers: Tony Wilson, Deroi Rose, Eisenhower
Williams & Adrian Fletcher

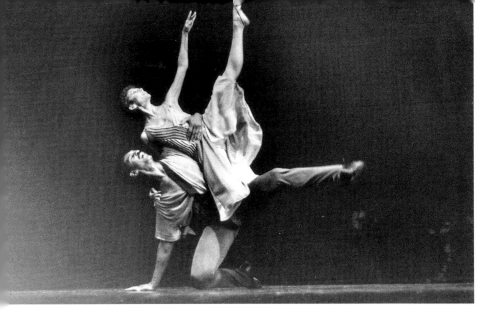

The National Dance Theatre Company, 1984
Dance: Recollections
Choreographer: Clive Thompson
Dancers: Clive Thompson & Melanie Graham

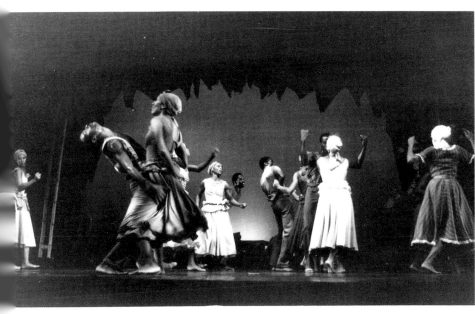

The National Dance Theatre Company, 1984
Dance: Gerrehbenta
Choreographer: Rex Nettleford
Dancers:The Company

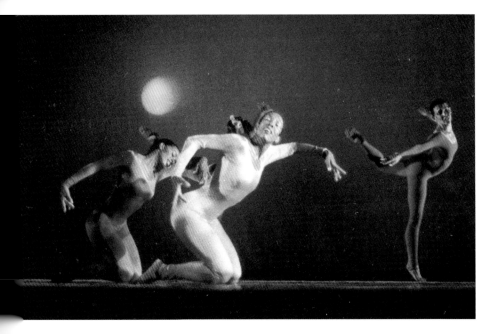

The National Dance Theatre Company, 1985
Dance: Islands
Choreographer: Rex Nettleford
Dancers: Denise Robinson, Gabrielle Harban &
Sandra Minott-Phillips

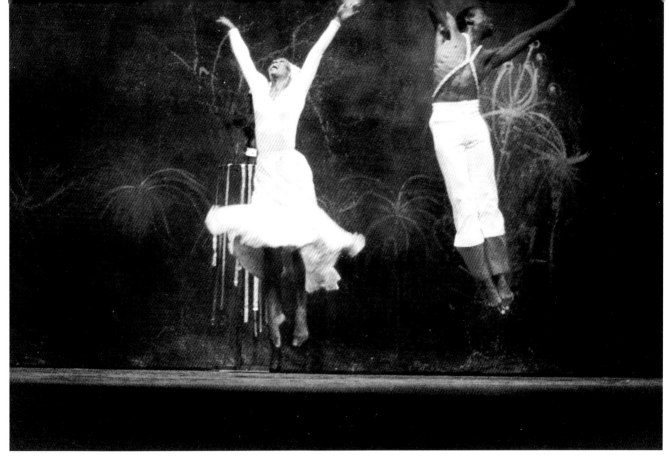

The National Dance Theatre Company, 1985 Dance: Celebrations Choreographer: Rex Nettleford Dancers: Gabrielle Harban & Christopher Morrison

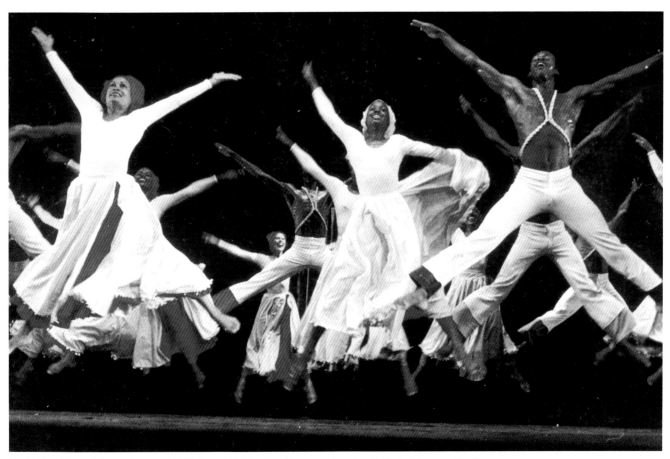

The National Dance Theatre Company, 1985 Dance: Celebrations Choreographer: Rex Nettleford Dancers: The Company

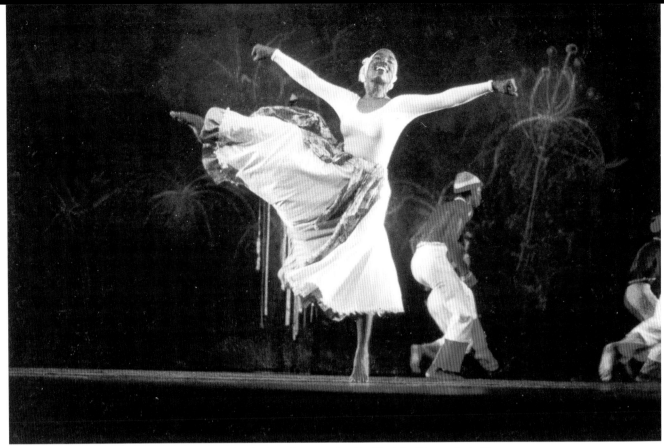

The National Dance Theatre Company, 1985 Dance: Celebrations Choreographer: Rex Nettleford Dancer: Paula Munroe

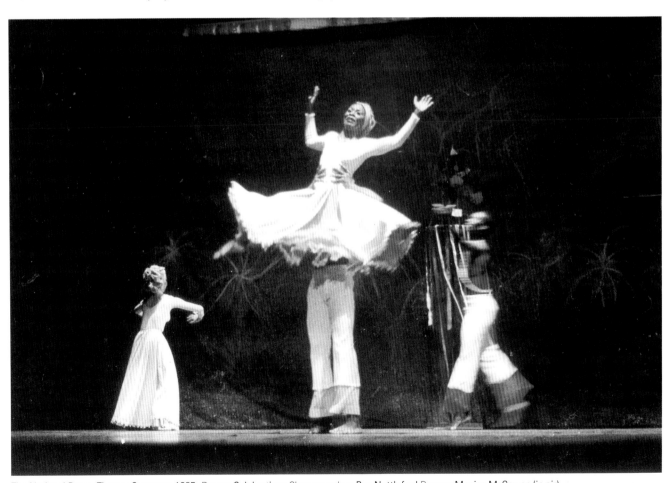

The National Dance Theatre Company, 1985 Dance: Celebrations Choreographer: Rex Nettleford Dancer: Monica McGowan (in air)

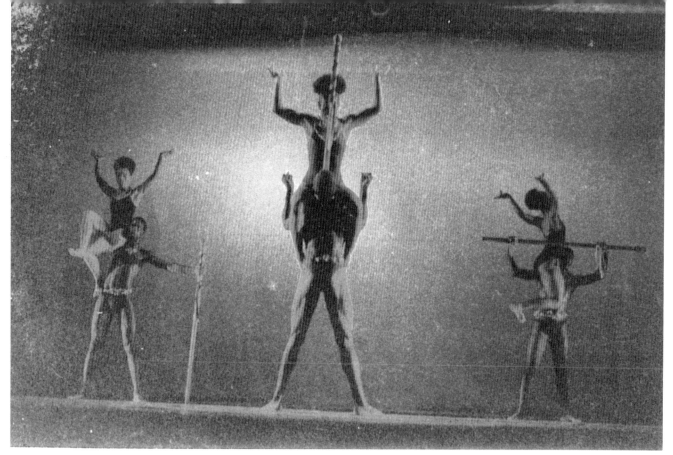

The National Dance Theatre Company, 1985 Dance: Sulkari Choreographer: Eduardo Rivera Dancers: Alaine Grant & Chris Morrison, Arlene Richards & Adrian Fletcher, Gabrielle Harban & Mark Ramsey

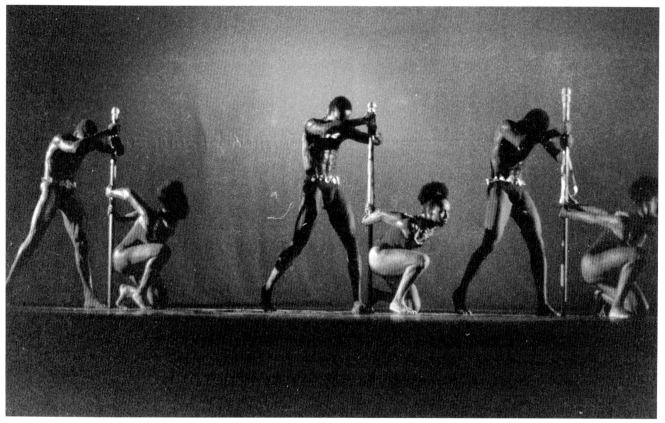

The National Dance Theatre Company, 1985 Dance: Sulkari Choreographer: Eduardo Rivera Dancers: Gabrielle Harban & Marik Ramsey, Alaine Grant & Chris Morrison, Arlene Richards & Adrian Fletcher

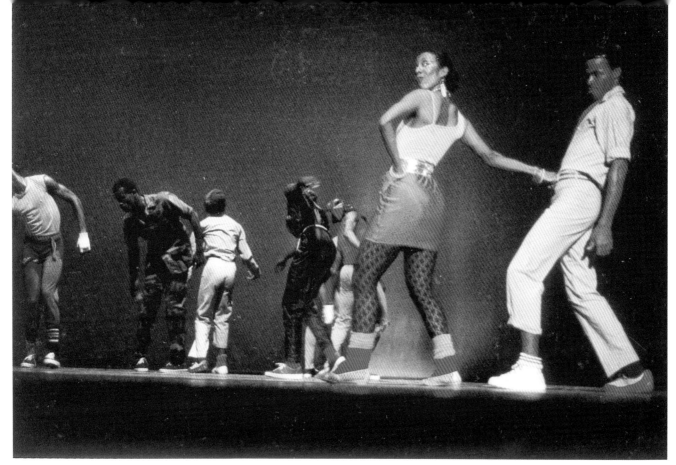

The National Dance Theatre Company, 1985 Dance: Puncie Choreographer: Rex Nettleford Dancers: Gabrielle Harban, Mark Ramsey & the Company

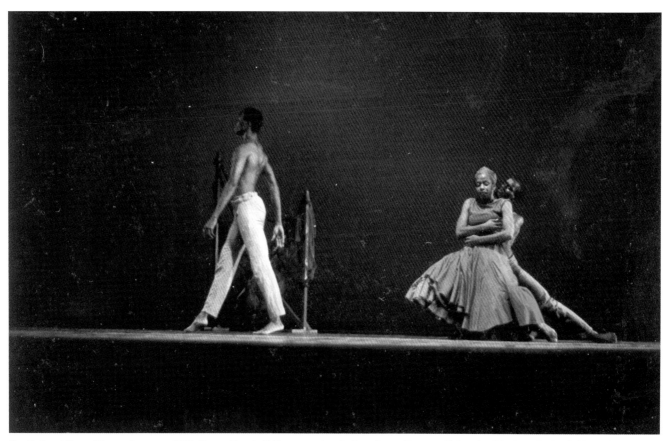

The National Dance Theatre Company, 1986 Dance: Treadmill Choreographer: Barbara Requa Dancers: Christopher Morrison, Denise Robinson & Monthy Williams

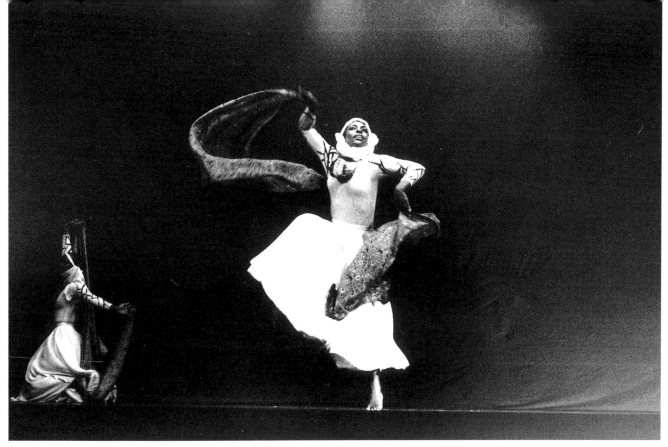

The National Dance Theatre Company, 1993 Dance: Interconnections Choreographer: Rex Nettleford Dancer: Denise Robinson (Ward Theatre)

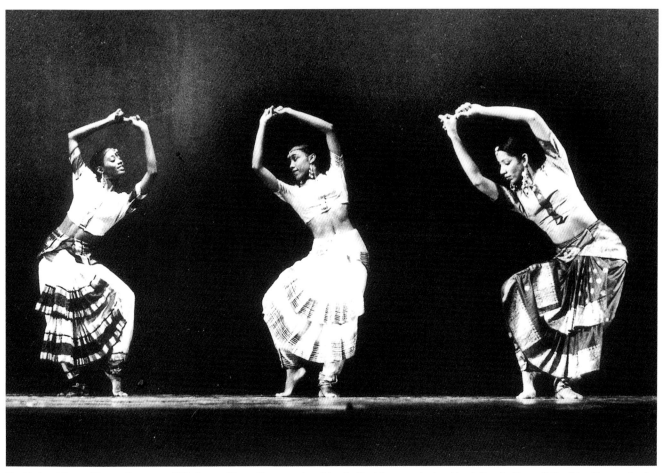

The National Dance Theatre Company, 1995 Dance: Mayur Choreographer: Meatha Soni Dancers: Andrea Lloyd, Natalie Chung & Staci-Lee Hassan-Fowles

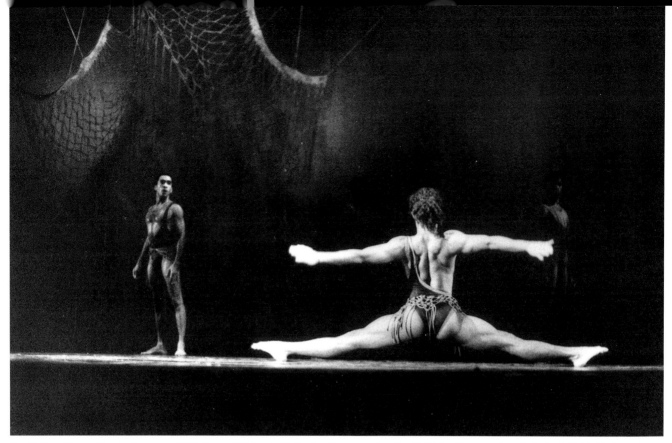

The National Dance Theatre Company, 1995 Dance: Spirits at a Gathering Choreographer: Rex Nettleford Dancers: Arsenio Andrade & Abeldo Gonsales

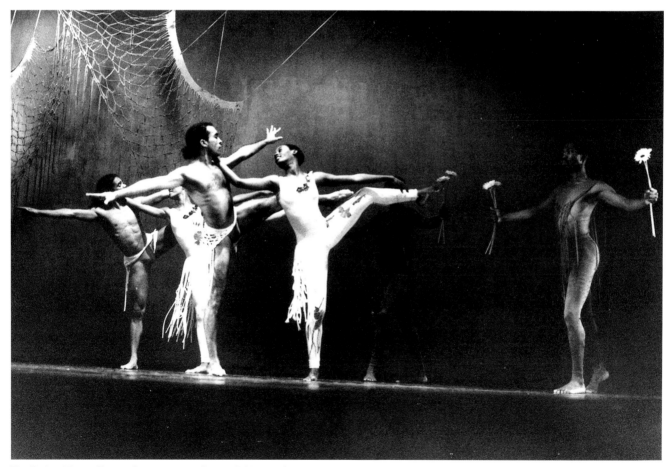

The National Dance Theatre Company, 1995 Dance: Spirits at a Gathering Choreographer: Rex Nettleford Dancers: Abeldo Gonsales; Arsenio Andrade, Andrea Lloyd & Milton Sterling

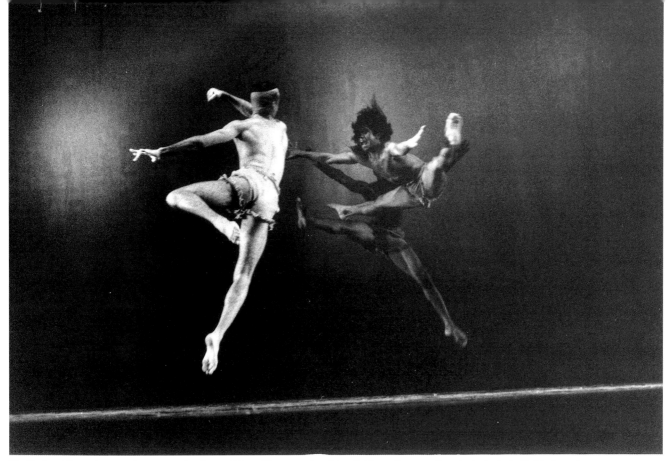

The National Dance Theatre Company, 1995 Dance: Tribute Choreographer: Eduardo Rivera Dancers: Arsenio Andrade & Abeldo Gonsales

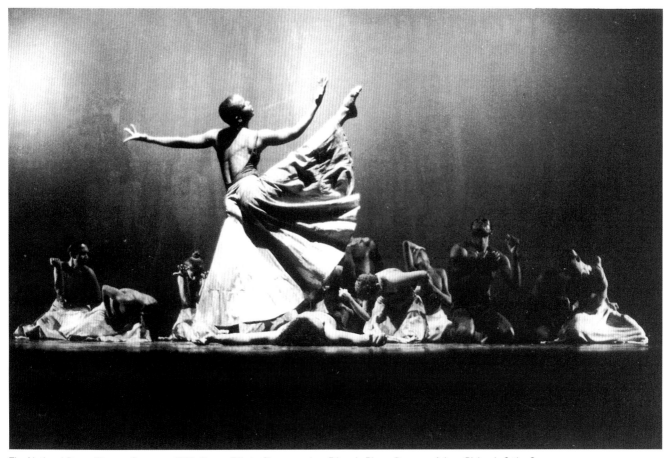

The National Dance Theatre Company, 1995 Dance: Tribute Choreographer: Eduardo Rivera Dancers: Arlene Richards & the Company

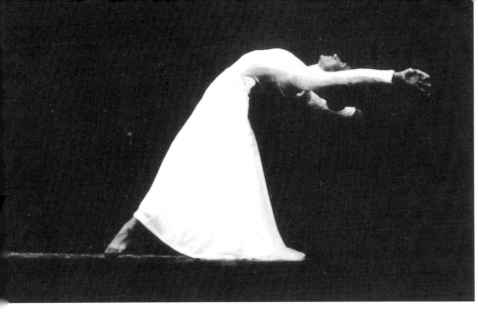

The National Dance Theatre Company, 1995
Dance: Vision
Choreographer: Clive Thompson
Dancer: Carole Orane Andrade

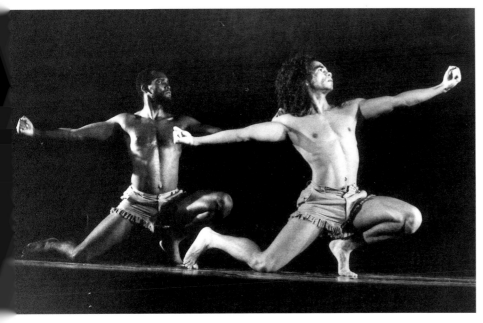

The National Dance Theatre Company, 1995
Dance: Tribute
Choreographer: Eduardo Rivera
Dancers: David Browne & Abeldo Gonsales

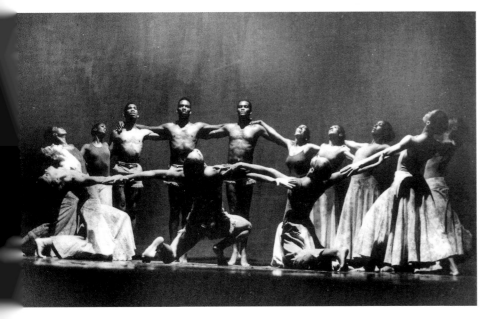

The National Dance Theatre Company, 1995
Dance: Tribute
Choreographer: Eduardo Rivera
Dancers: The Company

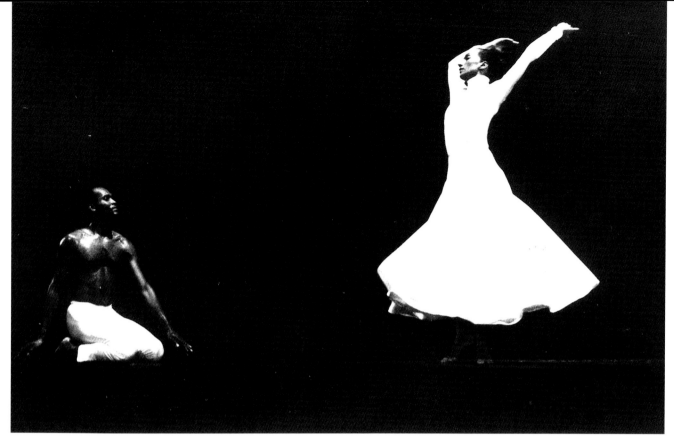

The National Dance Theatre Company, 1985 Dance: Vision Choreographer: Clive Thompson Dancers: David Browne & Carole Orane Andrade

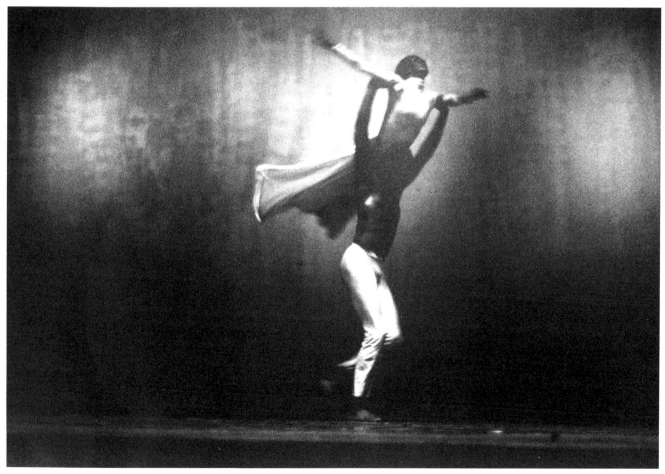

The National Dance Theatre Company, 1995 Dance: Vision Choreographer: Clive Thompson Dancers: David Browne & Carole Orane Andrade

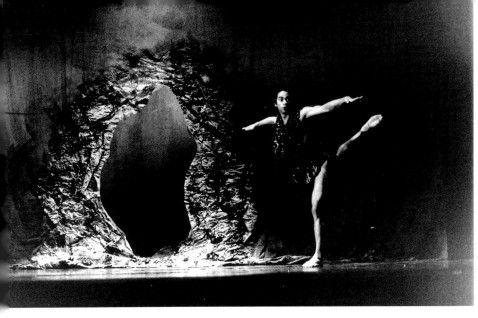

The National Dance Theatre Company, 1995
Dance: Rah
Choreographer: Arlene Richards
Dancer: Abeldo Gonsales

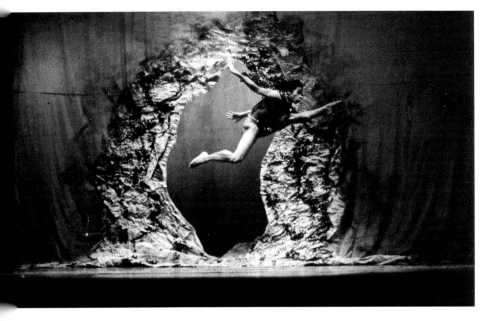

The National Dance Theatre Company, 1995
Dance: Rah
Choreographer: Arlene Richards
Dancer: Abeldo Gonsales

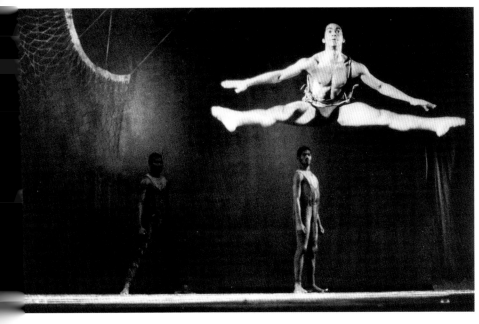

The National Dance Theatre Company, 1995
Dance: Spirits at a Gathering
Choreographer: Rex Nettleford
Dancers: Arsenio Andrade, David Browne,
Milton Sterling & Abeldo Gonsales

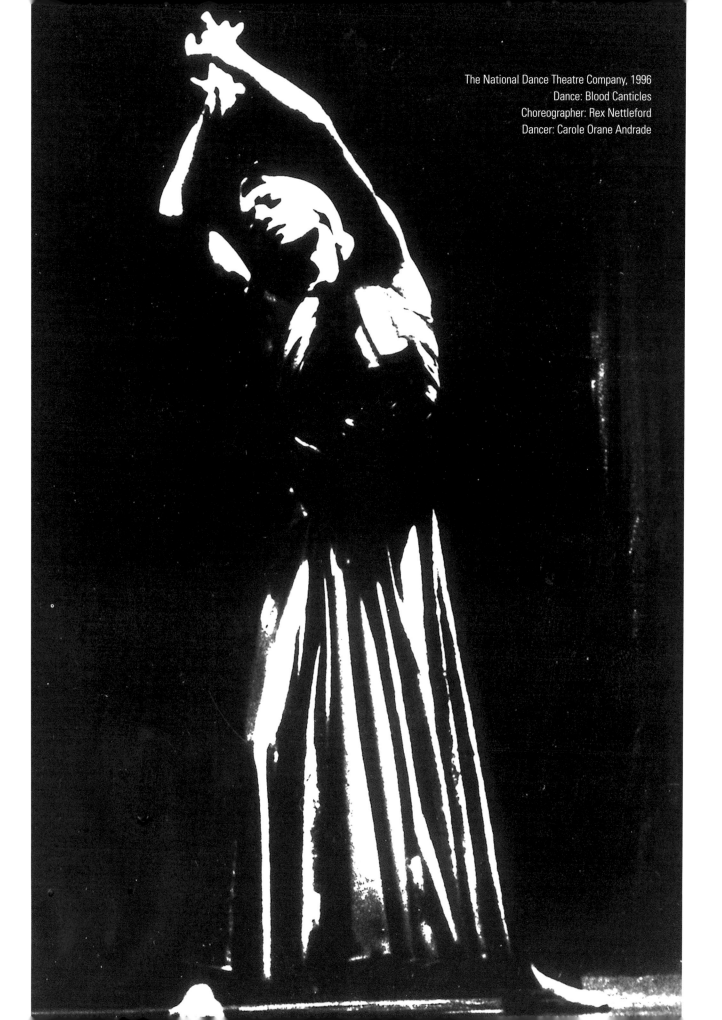

The National Dance Theatre Company, 1996
Dance: Blood Canticles
Choreographer: Rex Nettleford
Dancer: Carole Orane Andrade

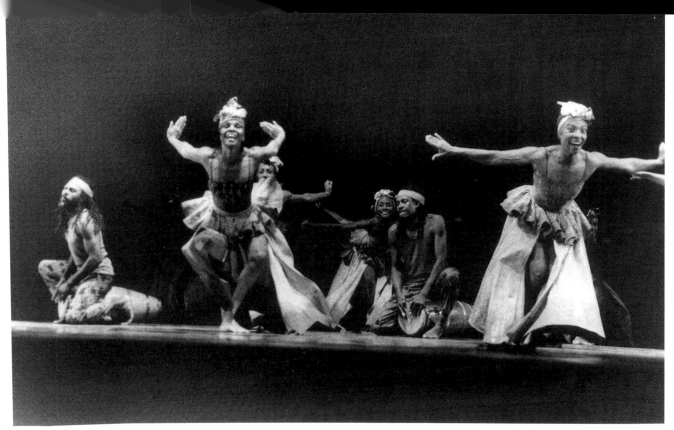

The National Dance Theatre Company, 1996 Dance: Drumscore Choreographer: Rex Nettleford Dancers: The Company, Billy Lawrence & Leaford McFarlane

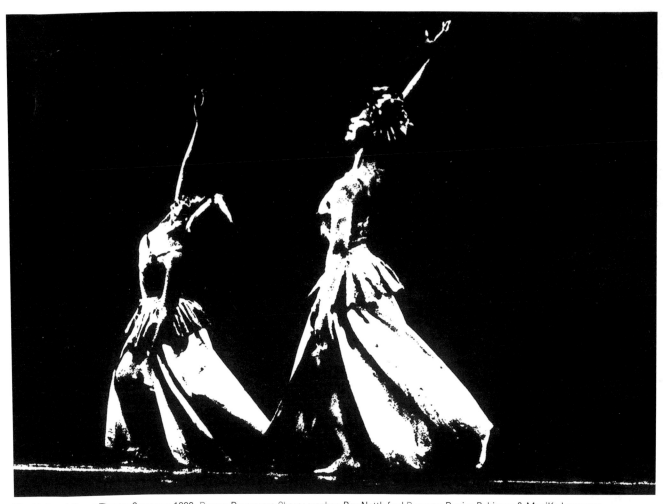

The National Dance Theatre Company, 1996 Dance: Drumscore Choreographer: Rex Nettleford Dancers: Denise Robinson & MoniKa Lawrence

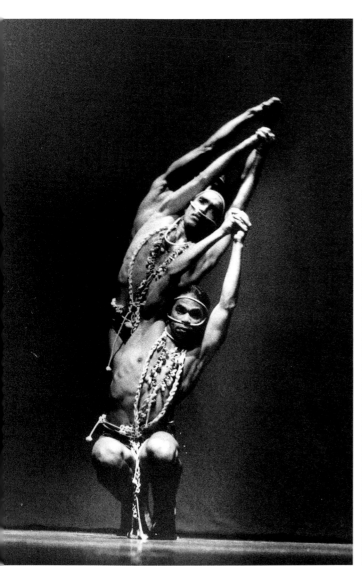

The National Dance Theatre Company, 1996
Dance: Blood Canticles
Choreographer: Rex Nettleford
Dancers: Abeldo Gonsales, Arsenio Andrade & Deroi Rose

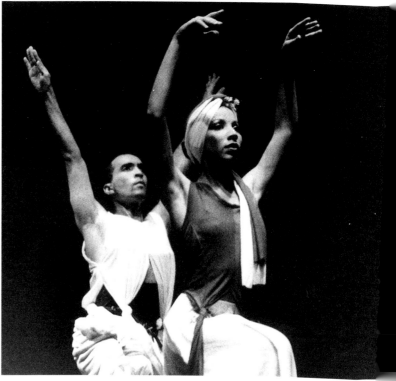

The National Dance Theatre Company, 1996
Dance: Blood Canticles
Choreographer: Rex Nettleford
Dancers: Arsenio Andrade & Staci-Lee Hassan-Fowles

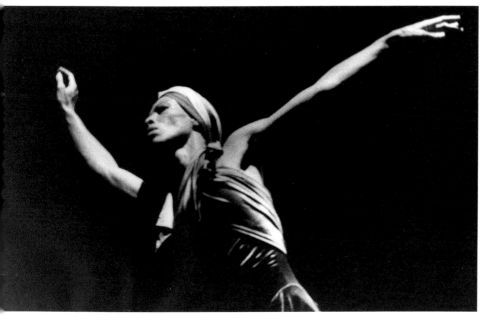

The National Dance Theatre Company, 1996
Dance: Blood Canticles
Choreographer: Rex Nettleford
Dancer: Alaine Grant

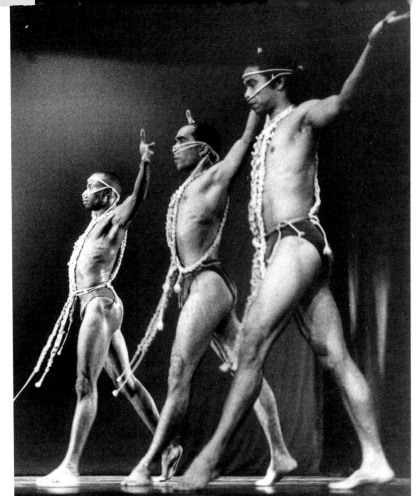

The National Dance Theatre Company, 1996
Dance: Blood Canticles
Choreographer: Rex Nettleford
Dancers: Deroi Rose, Arsenio Andrade & Abeldo Gonsales

The National Dance Theatre Company, 1996
Dance: He Watcheth
Choreographer: Milton Sterling
Dancers: Rolande Pryce, Kerry-Ann Henry,
Staci-Lee Hassan-Fowles & Natalie Chung

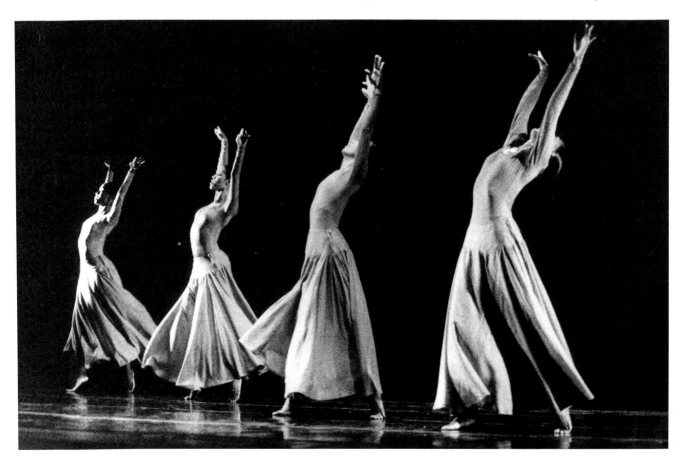

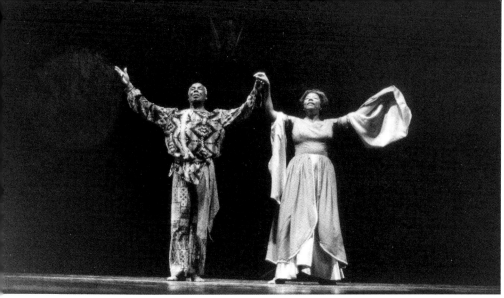

The National Dance Theatre Company, 1996
Dance: Kumina
Choreographer: Rex Nettleford
Dancers: Rex Nettleford & Pansy Hassan

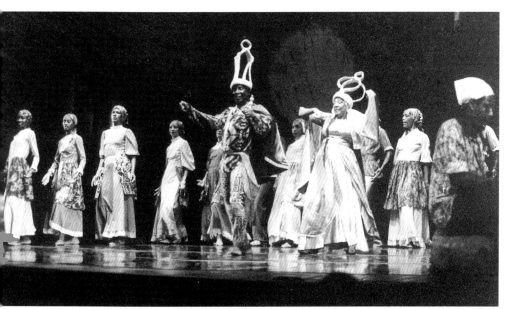

The National Dance Theatre Company, 1996
Dance: Kumina
Choreographer: Rex Nettleford
Dancers: Rex Nettleford, Pansy Hassan &
the Company

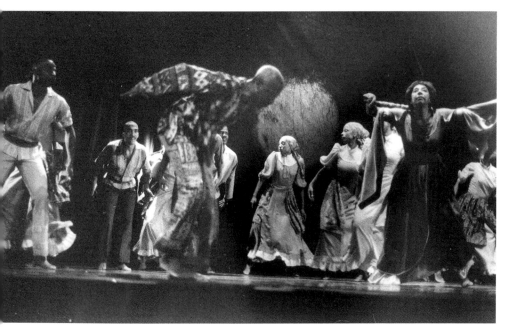

The National Dance Theatre Company, 1996
Dance: Kumina
Choreographer: Rex Nettleford
Dancers: Rex Nettleford, Pansy Hassan & the
Company

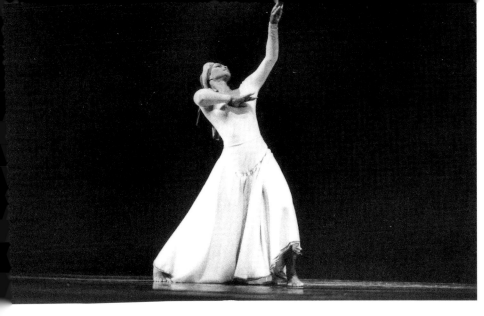

The National Dance Theatre Company, 1996
Dance: Cry of the Spirit
Choreographer: Gene Carson
Dancer: Arlene Richards

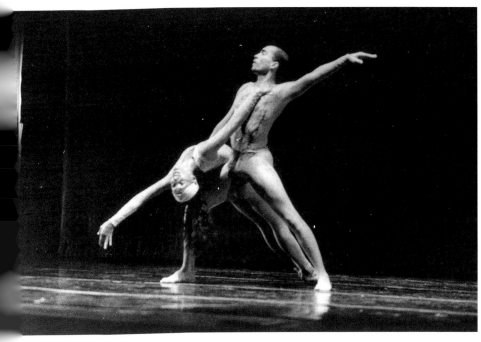

The National Dance Theatre Company, 1996
Dance: Earth Crisis
Choreographer: Arlene Richards
Dancers: Carol Orane Andrade & Arsenio Andrade

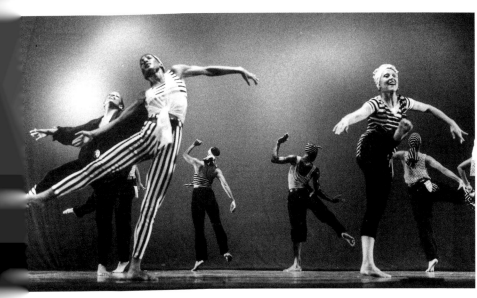

The National Dance Theatre Company, 1996
Dance: Bujurama
Choreographer: Rex Nettleford
Dancers: Denise Robinson, Carole Orane Andrade,
Melanie Graham & the Company

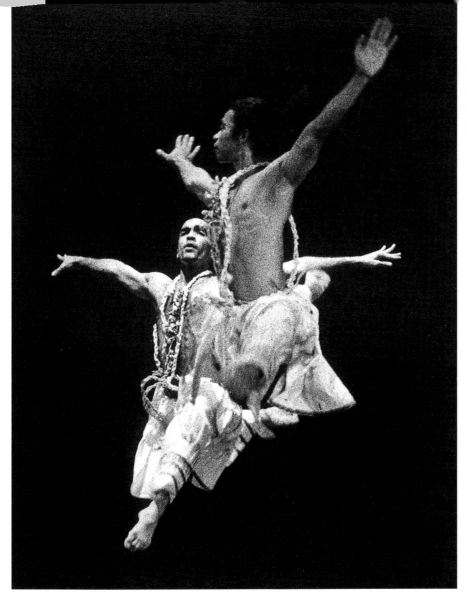

The National Dance Theatre Company, 1996
Dance: Blood Canticles
Choreographer: Rex Nettleford
Dancers: Arsenio Andrade & Abeldo Gonsales

The National Dance Theatre Company, 1996
Dance: Blood Canticles
Choreographer: Rex Nettleford
Dancers: The Company

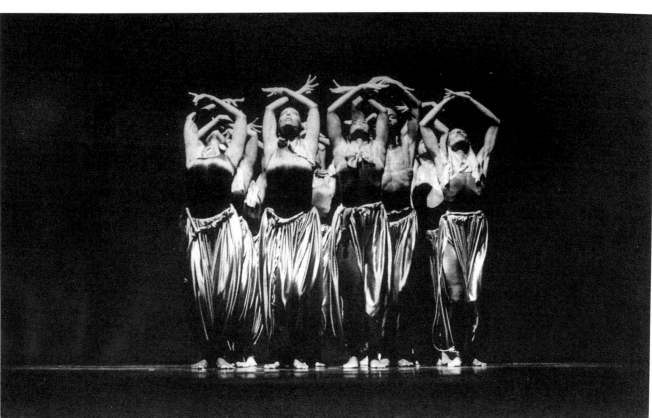

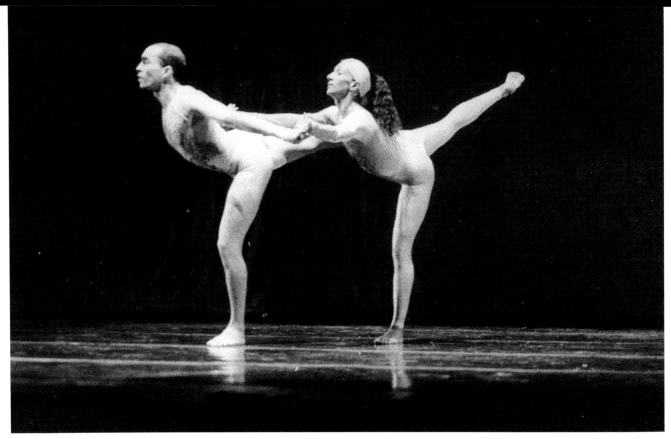

The National Dance Theatre Company, 1996 Dance: Earth Crisis Choreographer: Arlene Richards Dancers: Arsenio Andrade & Carole Orane Andrade

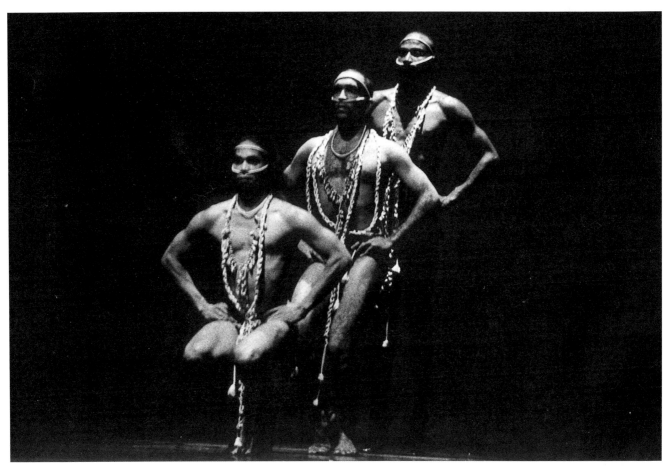

The National Dance Theatre Company, 1996 Dance: Blood Canticles Choreographer: Rex Nettleford Dancers: Abeldo Gonsales, Arsenio Anrade & Deroi Rose

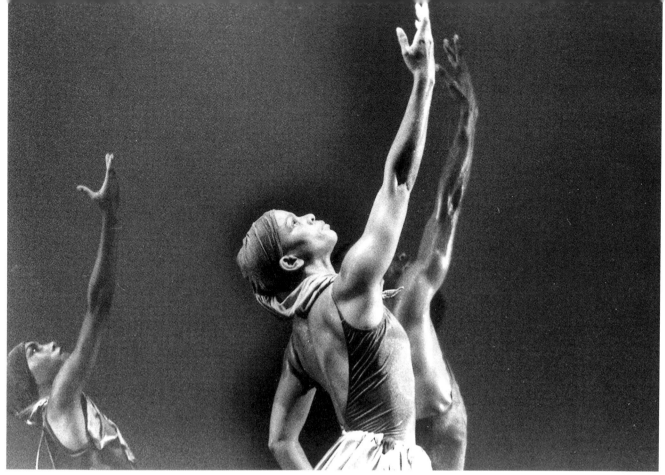

The National Dance Theatre Company, 1996 Dance: Blood Canticles Choreographer: Rex Nettleford Dancers: Natalie Chung, Arlene Richards & Deroi Rose

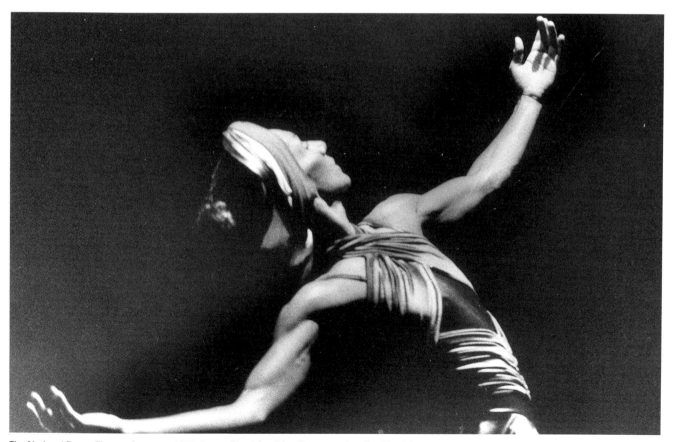

The National Dance Theatre Company, 1996 Dance: Blood Canticles Choreographer: Rex Nettleford Dancer: Carole Orane Andrade

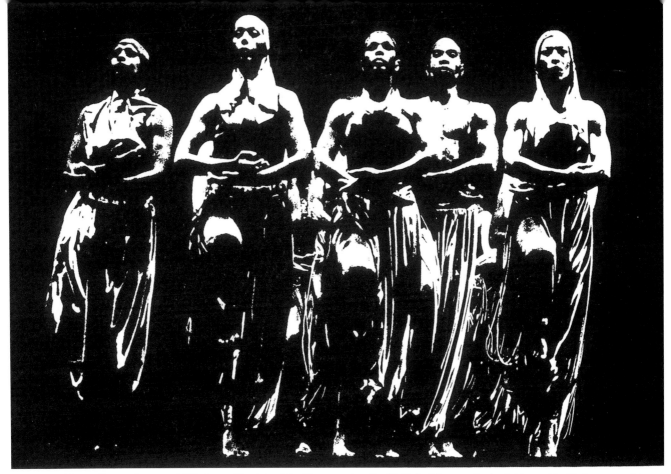

The National Dance Theatre Company, 1996 Dance: Blood Canticles Choreographer: Rex Nettleford Dancers: Denise Robinson, MoniKa Lawrence, Arlene Richards, Deroi Rose & Alaine Grant

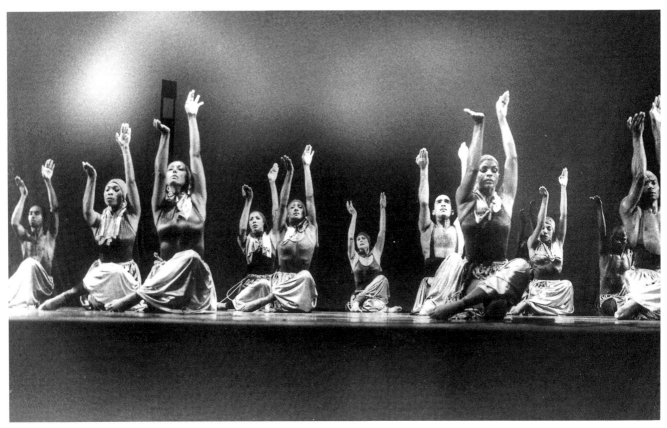

The National Dance Theatre Company, 1996 Dance: Blood Canticles Choreographer: Rex Nettleford Dancers: The Company

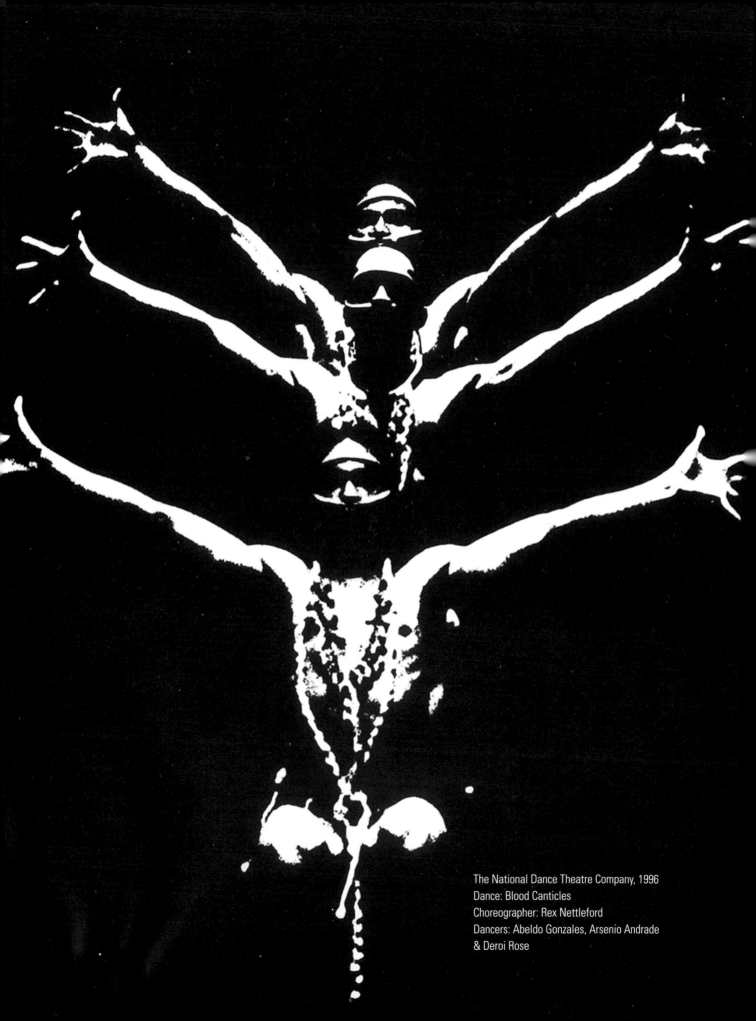

The National Dance Theatre Company, 1996
Dance: Blood Canticles
Choreographer: Rex Nettleford
Dancers: Abeldo Gonzales, Arsenio Andrade
& Deroi Rose

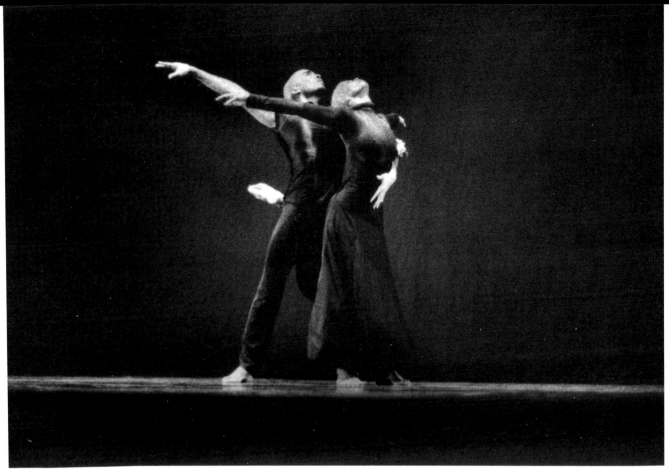

The National Dance Theatre Company, 1997 Dance: Steal Away Choreographer: Bert Rose Dancers: Arsenio Andrade & Arlene Richards

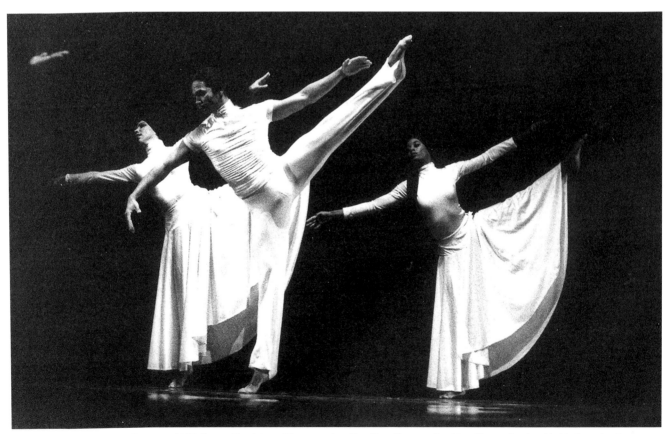

The National Dance Theatre Company, 1997 Dance: Steal Away Choreographer: Bert Rose Dancers: Staci-Lee Hassan-Fowles, Abeldo Gonsales &
Andrea Lloyd

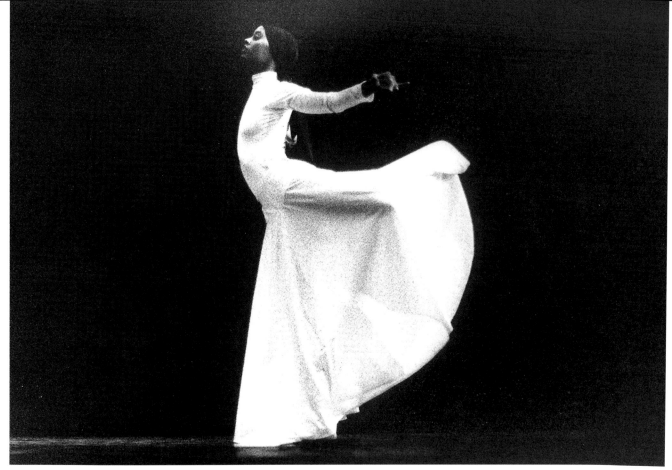

The National Dance Theatre Company, 1997 Dance: Steal Away Choreographer: Bert Rose Dancer: Andrea Lloyd

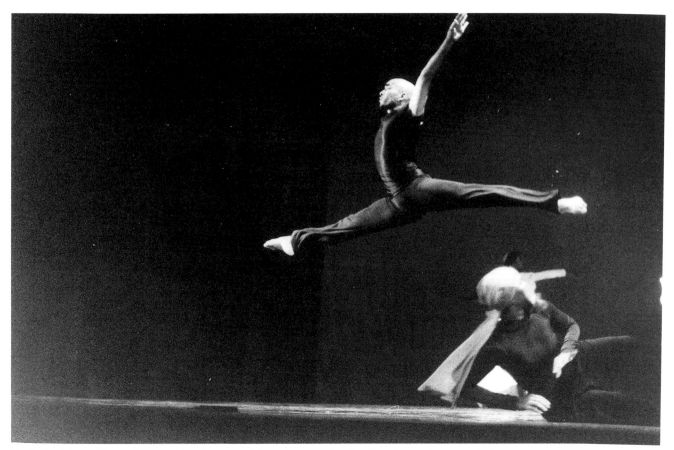

The National Dance Theatre Company, 1997 Dance: Steal Away Choreographer: Bert Rose Dancer: Arsenio Andrade

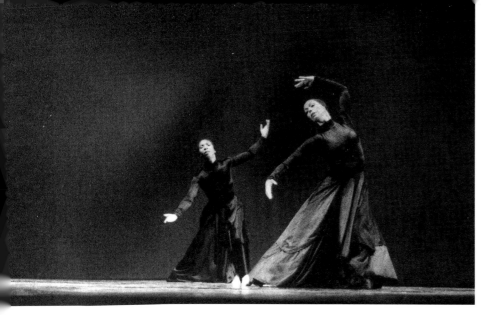

The National Dance Theatre, 1997
Dance: Tintinabulum
Choreographer: Rex Nettleford
Dancers: Allison Symes & MoniKa Lawrence

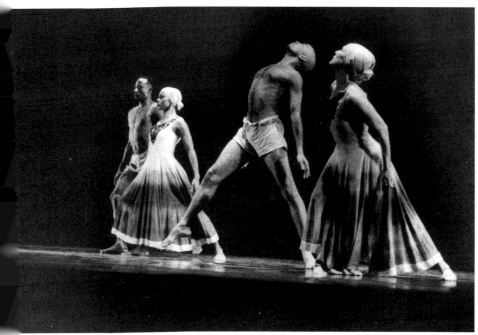

The National Dance Theatre Company, 1997
Dance: Tintinabulum
Choreographer: Rex Nettleford
Dancers: Deroi Rose, Arlene Richards, Arsenio
Andrade & Melanie Graham

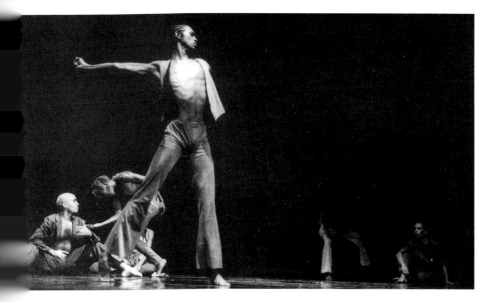

The National Dance Theatre
Company, 1997
Dance: Voices
Choreographer: Arlene Richards
Dancers: Arsenio Andrade, Andrea Lloyd, Christopher
Walker & Alaine Grant

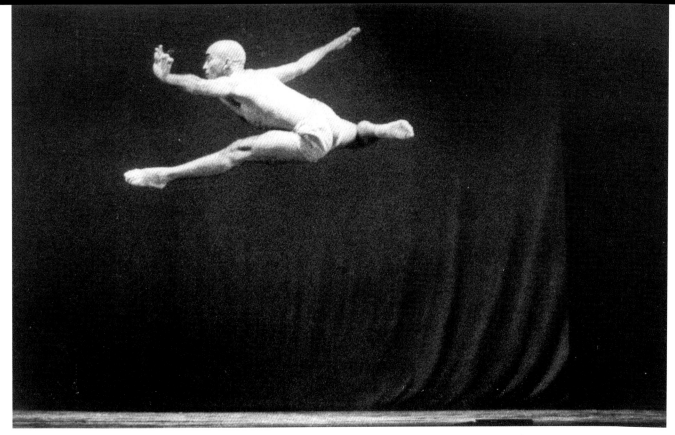

The National Dance Theatre Company, 1997   Dance: Tintinabulum Choreographer: Rex Nettleford Dancer: Arsenio Andrade

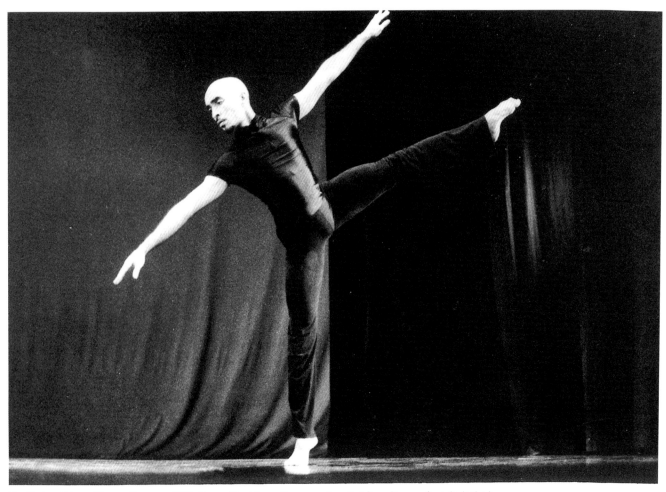

The National Dance Theatre Company, 1997   Dance: Steal Away Choreographer: Bert Rose Dancer: Arsenio Andrade

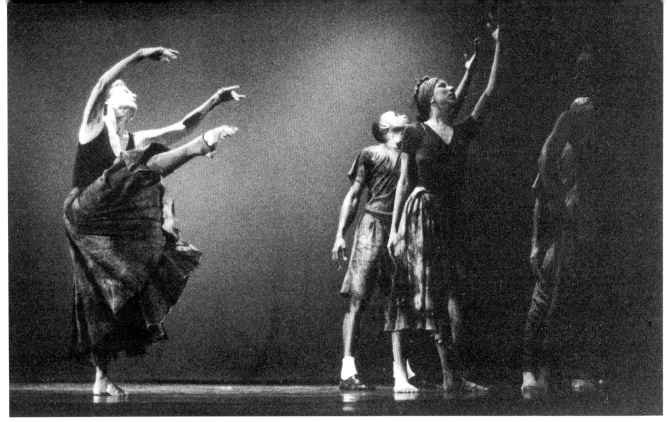

The National Dance Theatre Company, 1997 Dance: Selah Choreographer: MoniKa Lawrence Dancers: Melanie Graham, Deroi Rose & Staci-Lee Hassan-Fowles

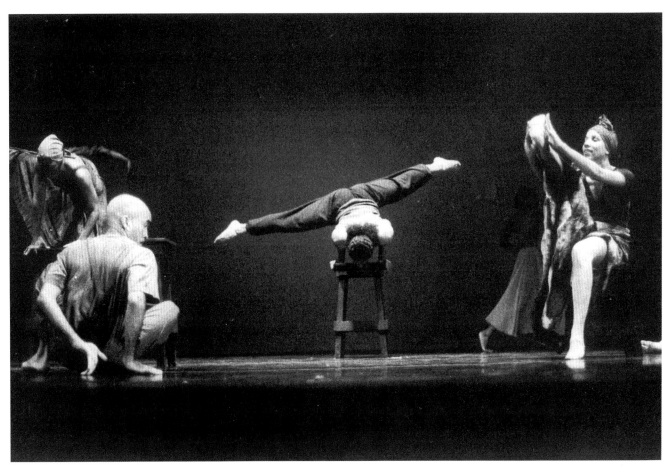

The National Dance Theatre Company, 1997 Dance: Selah Choreographer: MoniKa Lawrence Dancers: Arsenio Andrade, Abeldo Gonzales & Staci-Lee Hassan-Fowles

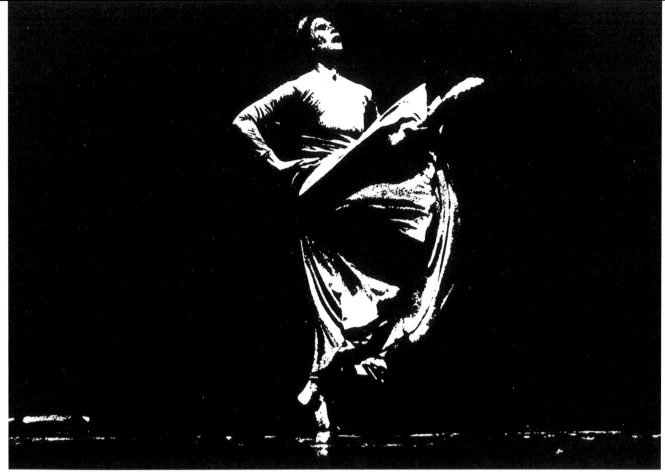

The National Dance Theatre Company, 1997 Dance: Cry of the Spirit Choreographer: Gene Carson Dancer: Melanie Graham

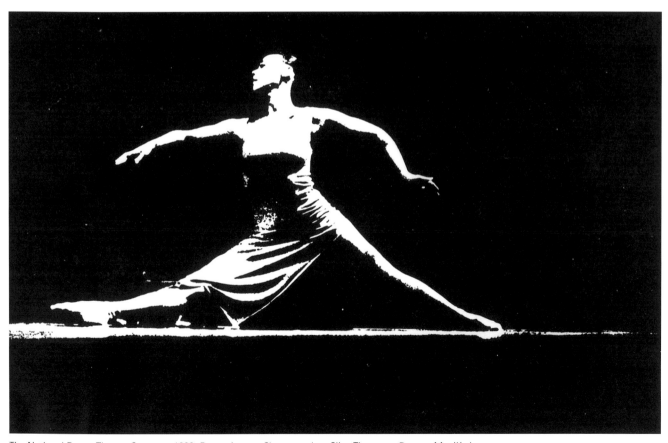

The National Dance Theatre Company, 1998 Dance: Images Choreographer: Clive Thompson Dancer: MoniKa Lawrence

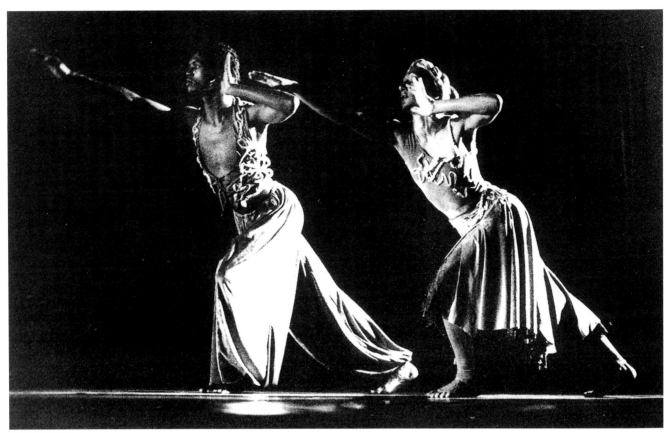

The National Dance Theatre Company, 1998 Dance: Images Choreographer: Clive Thompson Dancers: Christopher Walker & Carole Orane Andrade

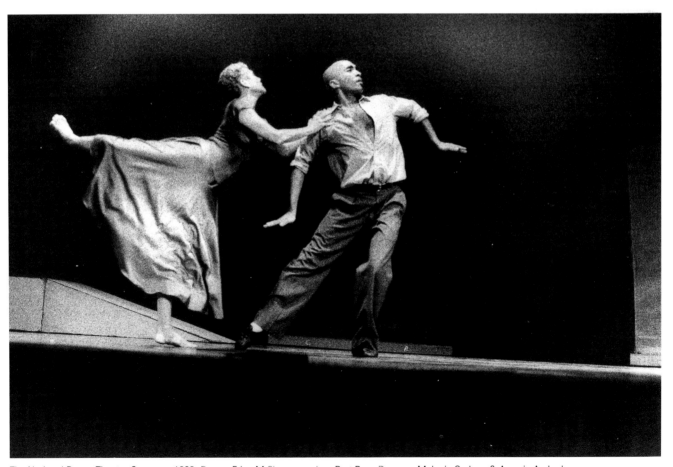

The National Dance Theatre Company, 1998 Dance: Edna M Choreographer: Bert Rose Dancers: Melanie Graham & Arsenio Andrade

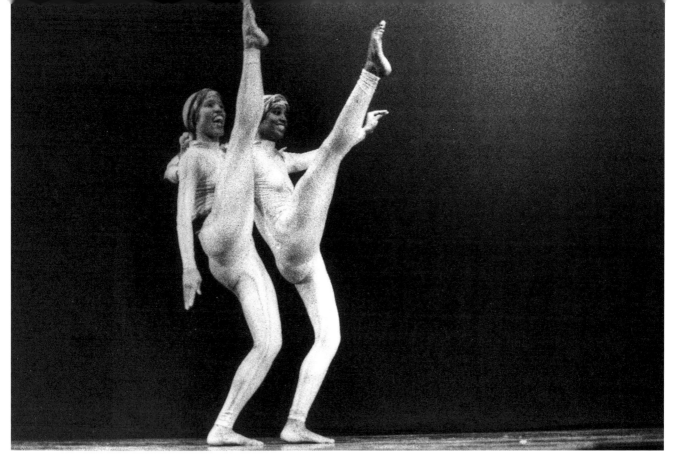

The National Dance Theatre Company, 1998 Dance: Side By Side Choreographer: Arlene Richards Dancers: Kerry Ann Henry & Andrea Lloyd

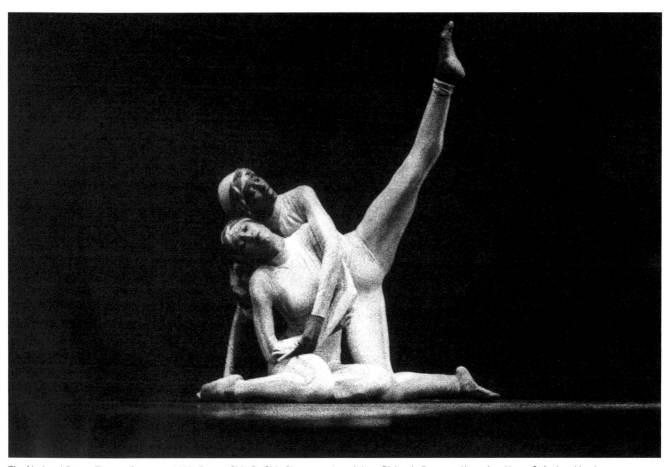

The National Dance Theatre Company, 1998 Dance: Side By Side Choreographer: Arlene Richards Dancers: Kerry Ann Henry & Andrea Lloyd

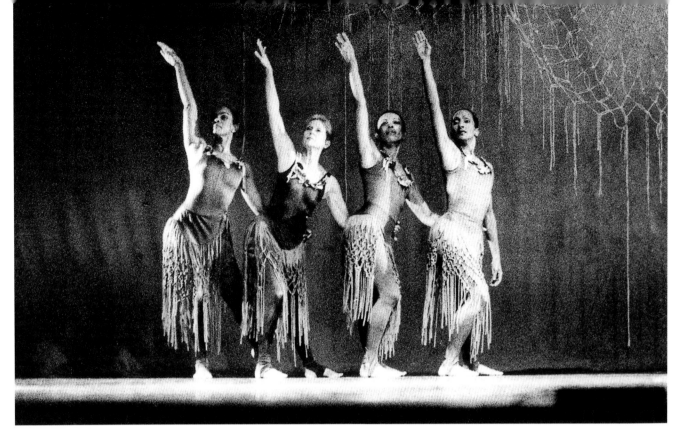

The National Dance Theatre Company, 1998 Dance: Spirits at a Gathering Choreographer: Rex Nettleford Dancers: Arlene Richards, Melanie Graham, Alaine Grant & Carole Orane Andrade

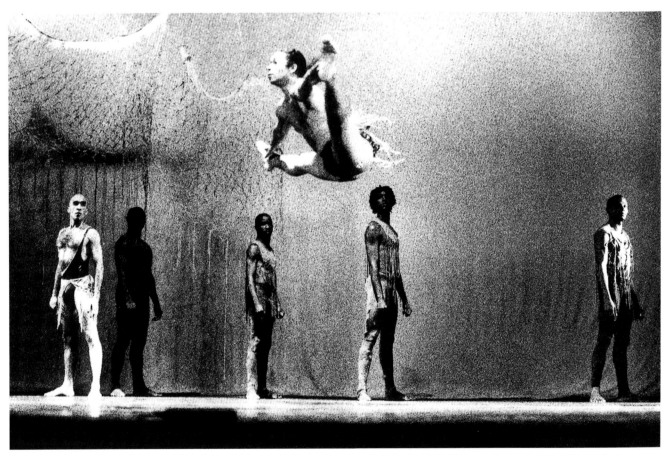

The National Dance Theatre Company, 1998 Dance: Spirits at a Gathering Choreographer: Rex Nettleford Dancers: Abeldo Gonsales, Arsenio Andrade, Keith Fagan, Franklyn Bryson, Chris Walker & Deroi Rose (background)

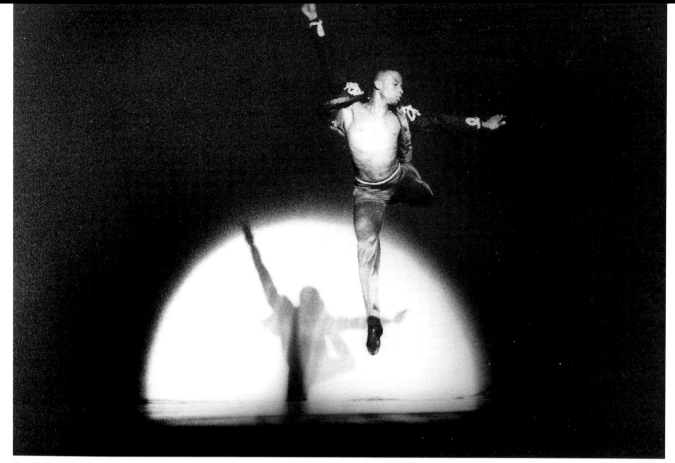

The National Dance Theatre Company, 1998 Dance: The Edge Choreographer: MoniKa Lawrence Dancer: Deroi Rose

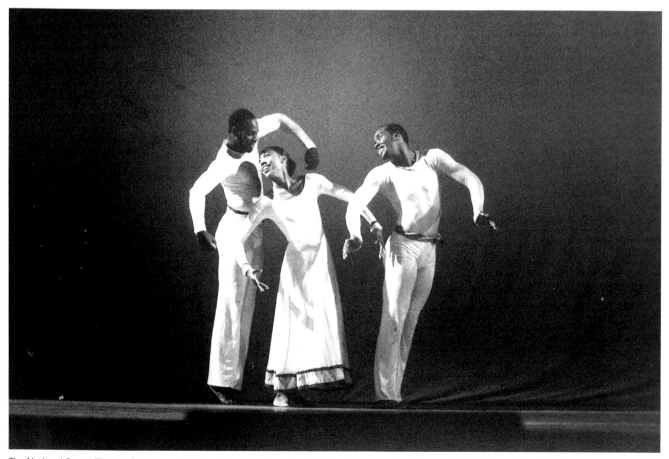

The National Dance Theatre Company, : Hold Fast Choreographer: Rex Nettleford Dancers: Kevin Moore, Natalie Chung & David Blake

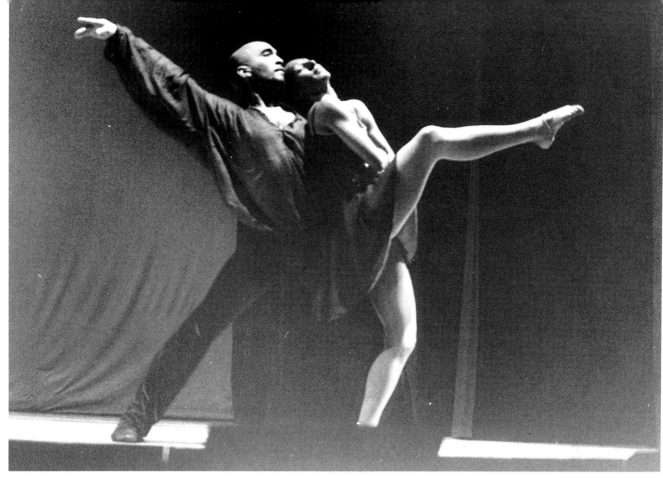

The National Dance Theatre Company, 2001 Dance : Footprints Choreographer: Arsenio Andrade Dancers: Arsenio Andrade & Carole Orane Andrade

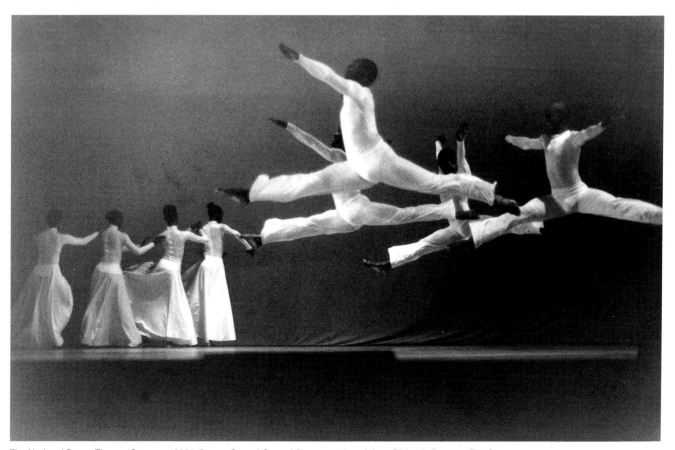

The National Dance Theatre Company, 2001 Dance: Sacred Ground Choreographer: Arlene Richards Dancers: The Company

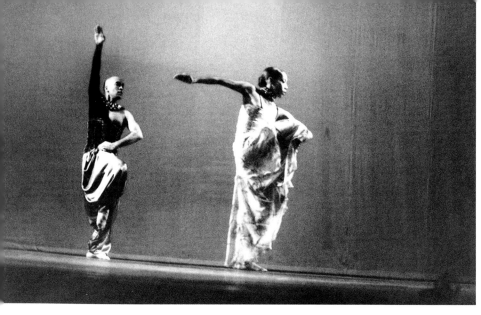

The National Dance Theatre Company, 2002
Dance: Michezo
Choreographer: Tony Wilson
Dancers: Arsenio Andrade & Natalie Chung

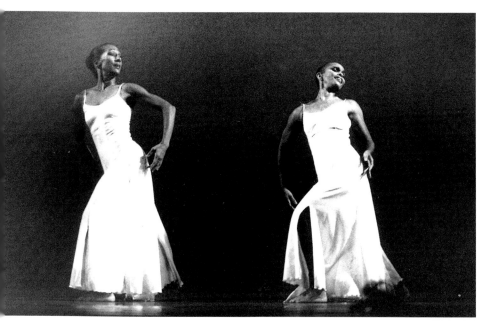

The National Dance Theatre Company, 2002
Dance: Cave's End
Choreographer: Rex Nettleford
Dancers: Carole Orane Andrade & Arlene Richards

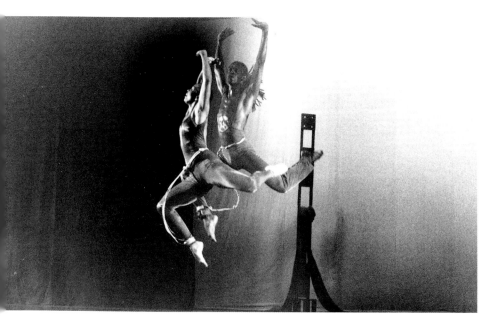

The National Dance Theatre Company, 2002
Dance: Blood Canticles
Choreographer: Rex Nettleford
Dancers: Arlene Richards & Christopher Walker

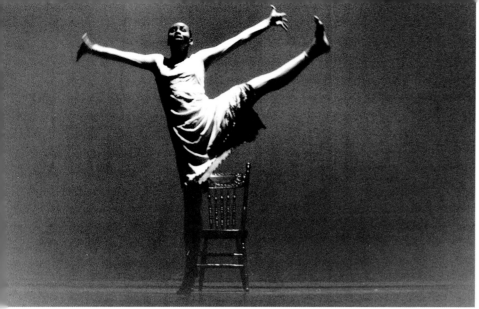

The National Dance Theatre Company, 2002
Dance: Flashback 'Fear'
Choreographer: conceived by Arlene Richards (original)
choreography Joyce Campbell
Dancer: Keita-Marie Chamberlain

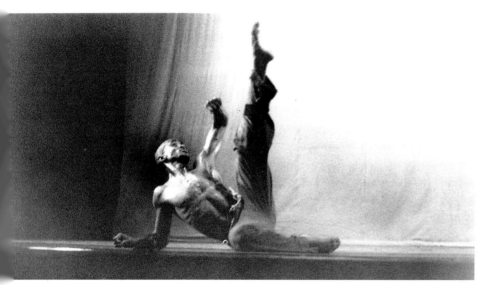

The National Dance Theatre Company, 2002
Dance: Flashback 'Street People'
Choreographer: conceived by Arlene Richards (original)
choreography Rex Nettleford
Dancer: Marlon Simms

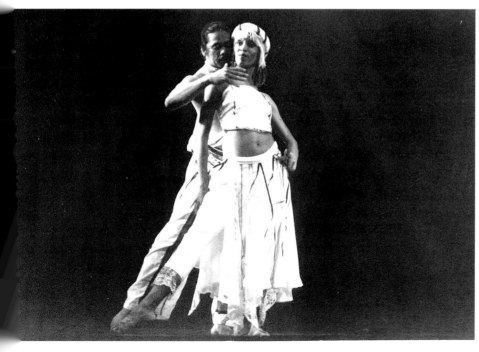

The National Dance Theatre Company, 2002
Dance: Brazilian Ode
Choreographer: Rex Nettleford
Dancers: Abeldo Gonsales & Kerry Ann Henry

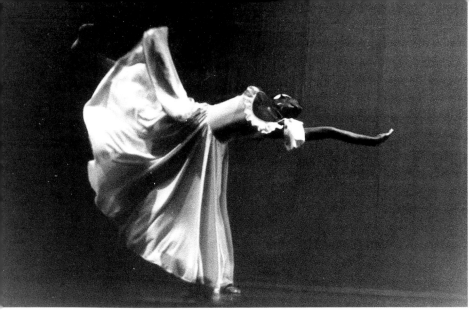

The National Dance Theatre Company, 2002
Dance: Incantation
Choreographer: Jean Guy Saintus
Dancer: Kerry Ann Henry

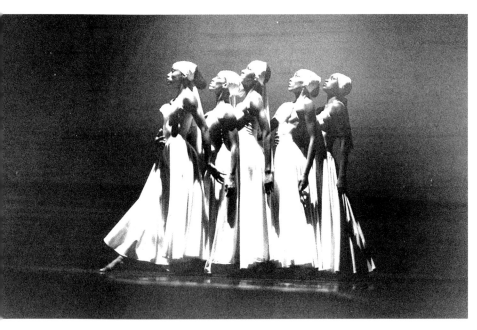

The National Dance Theatre Company, 2002
Dance: Incantation
Choreographer: Jean Guy Saintus
Dancers: Debroah Powell, Kerry-Ann Henry, Kafi Jones,
Natalie Chung & Keita-Marie Chamberlain

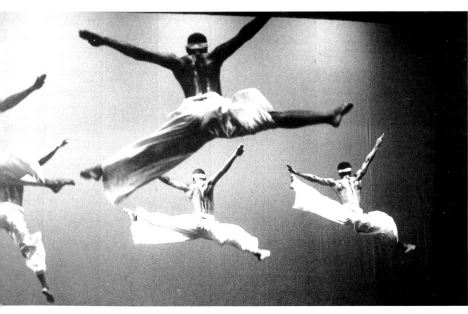

The National Dance Theatre Company, 2002
Dance: Incantation
Choreographer: Jean Guy Saintus
Dancers: Kevin Moore, Germaine Rowe & Mark Phinn

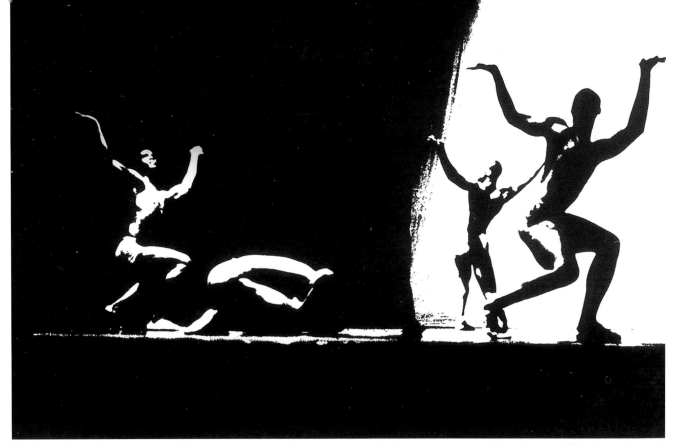

The National Dance Theatre Company, 2002 Dance: Incantation Choreographer: Jean Guy Saintus Dancers: Mark Phinn, Germaine Rowe, Marlon Simms & Kevin Moore

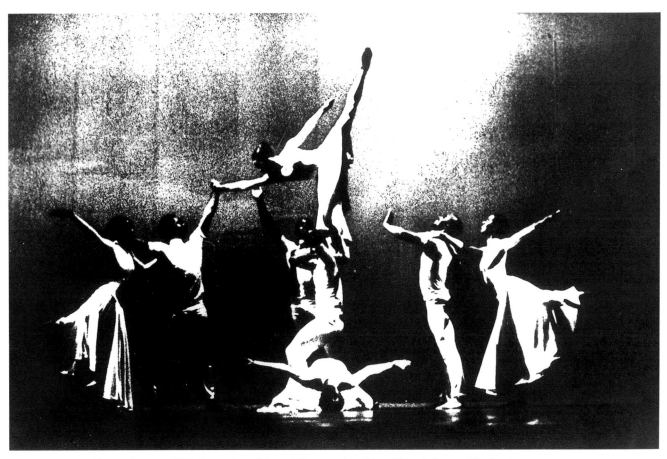

The National Dance Theatre Company, 2002 Dance: Sacred Ground Choreographer: Arlene Richards Dancers: The Company

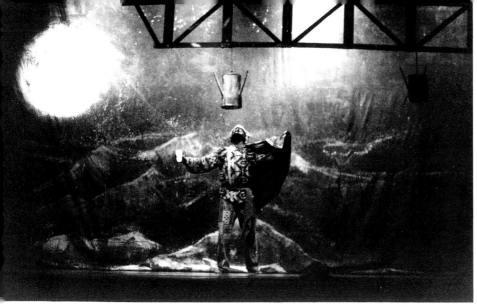

The National Dance Theatre Company, 2002
Dance: Kumina
Choreographer: Rex Nettleford
Dancer: Rex Nettleford

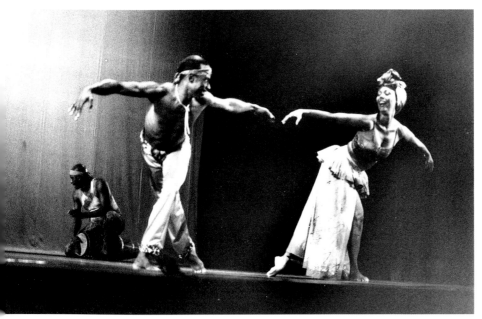

The National Dance Theatre Company, 2002
Dance: Drumscore
Choreographer: Rex Nettleford
Dancers: Deroi Rose & MoniKa Lawrence

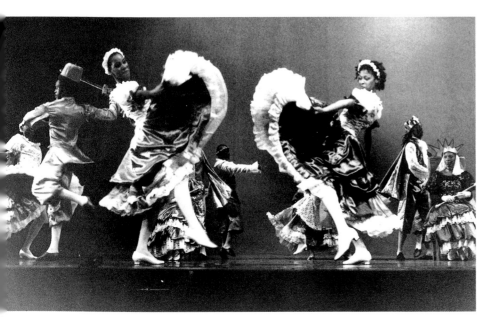

The National Dance Theatre Company, 2002
Dance: Bruckins
Choreographers: Joyce Campbell & Barry Moncrieffe
Dancers: The Company

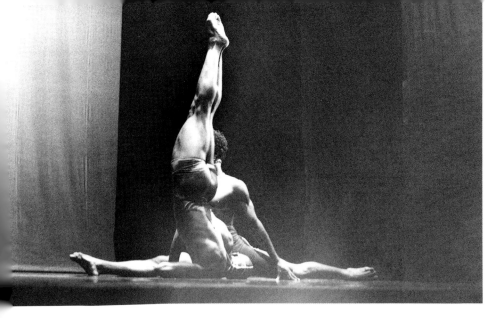

The National Dance Theatre Company, 2002
Dance: Millenial Beings
Choreographer: Marlon Simms
Dancers: Marlon Simms & Mark Phinn

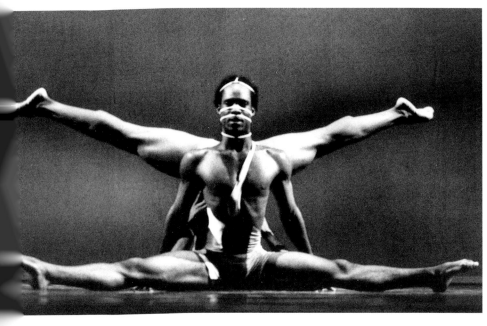

The National Dance Theatre Company, 2002
Dance: Millenial Beings
Choreographer: Marlon Simms
Dancers: Mark Phinn & Marlon Simms

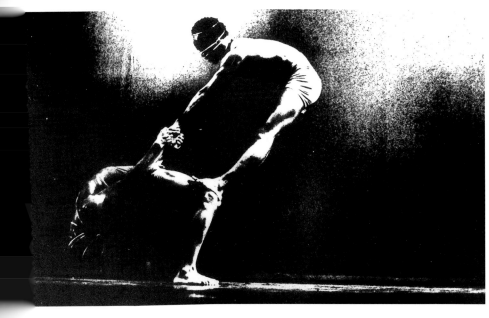

The National Dance Theatre Company, 2002
Dance: Millenial Beings
Choreographer: Marlon Simms
Dancers: Marlon Simms & Mark Phinn

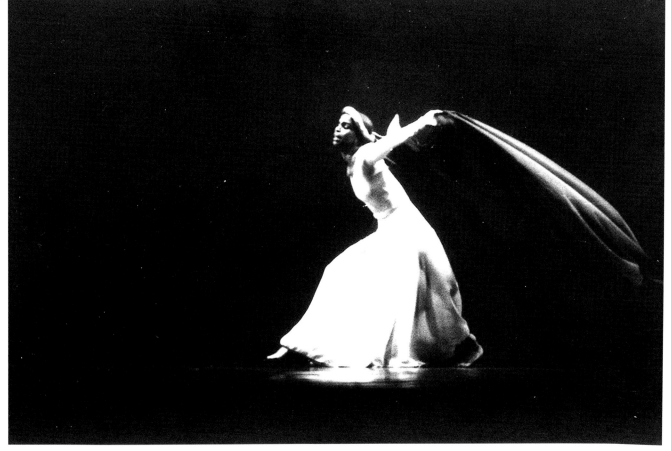

The National Dance Theatre Company, 2002 Dance: Cry of the Spirit Choreographer: Gene Carson Dancer: Arlene Richards

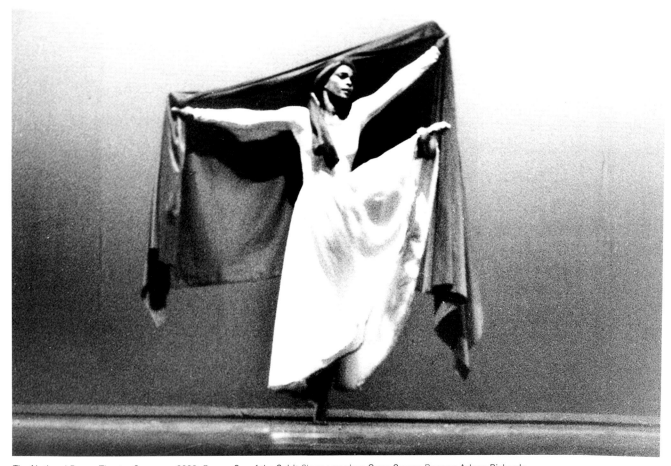

The National Dance Theatre Company, 2002 Dance: Cry of the Spirit Choreographer: Gene Carson Dancer: Arlene Richards

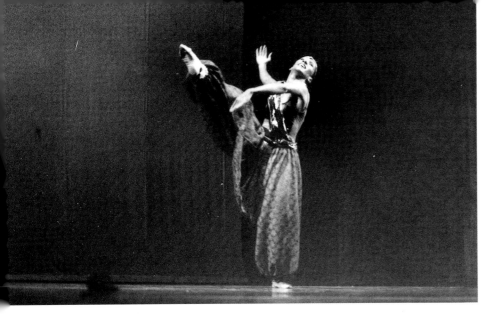

The National Dance Theatre Company, 2002
Dance: Cross Currents
Choreographer: MoniKa Lawrence
Dancer: Carole Orane Andrade

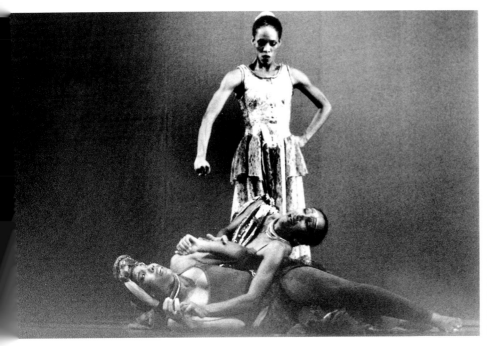

The National Dance Theatre Company, 2002
Dance: Cross Currents
Choreographer: MoniKa Lawrence
Dancers: Natalie Chung, Carole Orane Andrade &
Kerry-Ann Henry

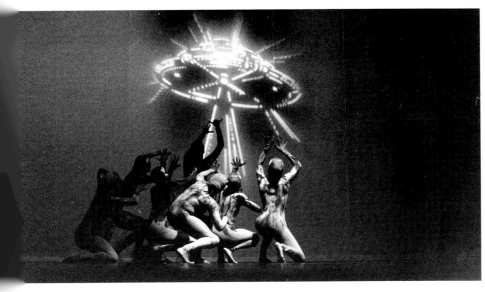

The National Dance Theatre Company, 2002
Dance: Cocoon
Choreographer: Arlene Richards
Dancers: The Company

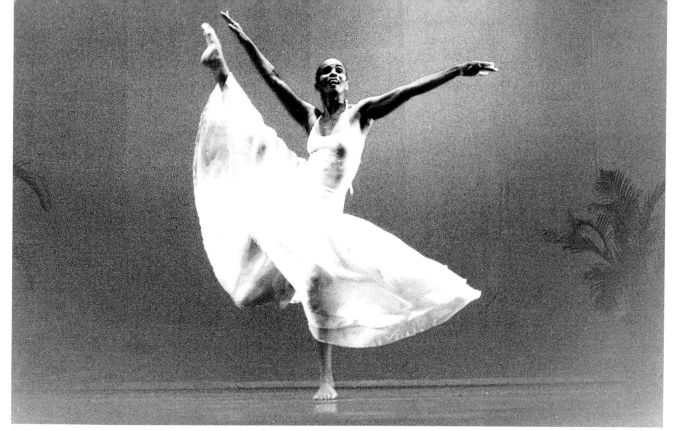

The National Dance Theatre Company, 2002   Dance: Phases of Three Moons Choreographer: Clive Thompson Dancer: Arlene Richards

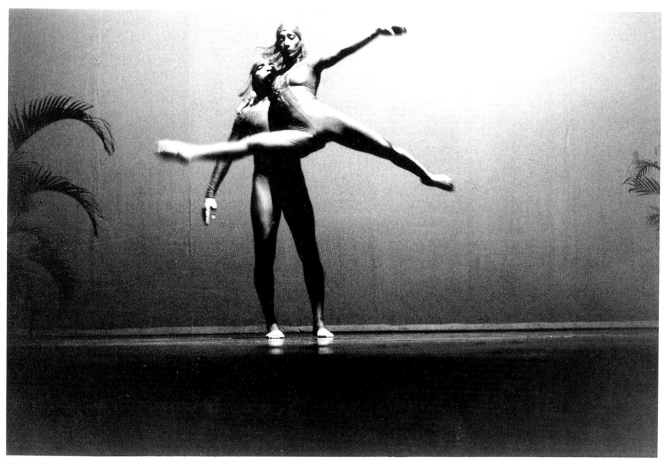

The National Dance Theatre Company, 2002   Dance: Phases of Three Moons Choreographer: Clive Thompson Dancers: Carole Orane Andrade &
Arsenio Andrade

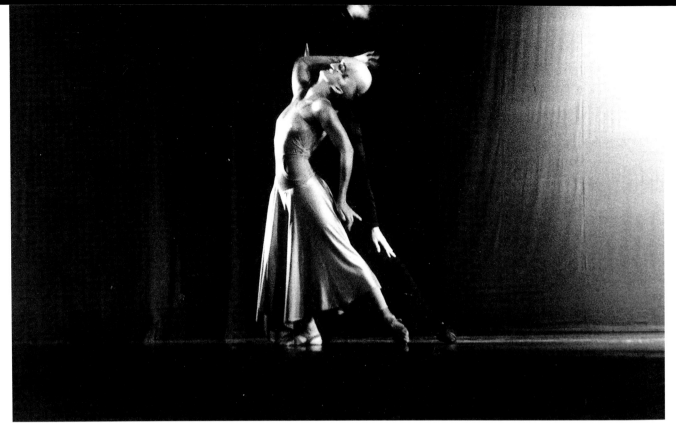

The National Dance Theatre Company, 2002 Dance: Legacy of the Duke Choreographer: Clive Thompson Dancers: Arlene Richards & Arsenio Andrade

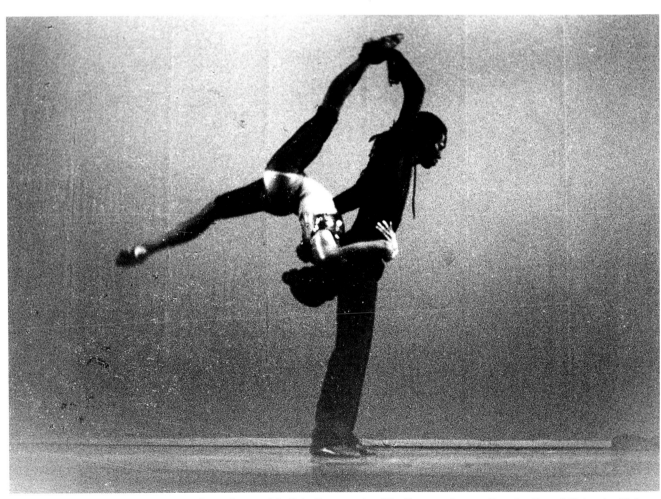

The National Dance Theatre Company, 2002 Dance: Legacy of the Duke Choreographer: Clive Thompson Dancers: Kerry-Ann Henry & Christopher Walker

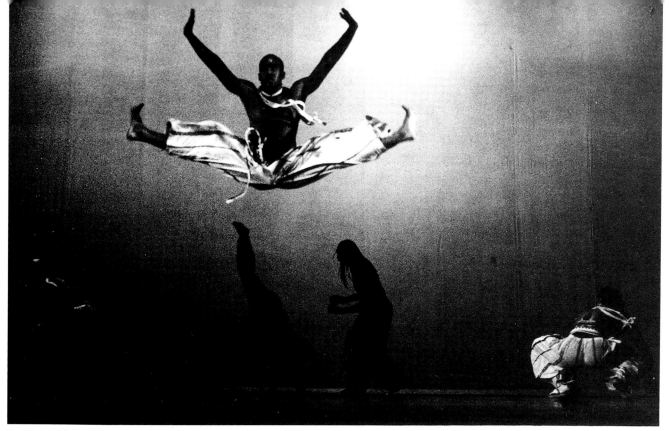

The National Dance Theatre Company, 2002 Dance: Brazilian Ode Choreographer: Rex Nettleford Dancer: David Blake (in air)

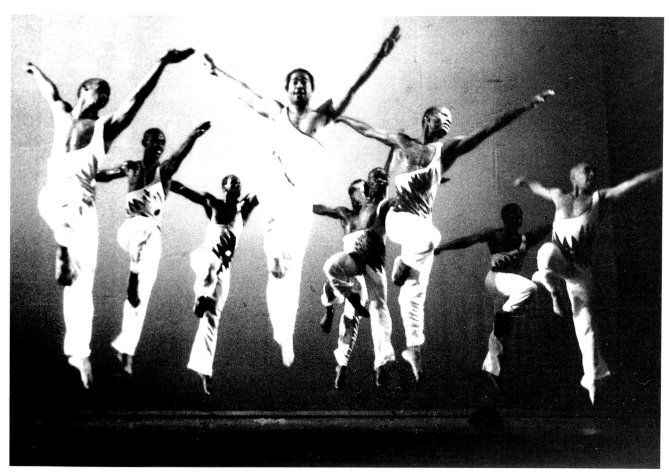

The National Dance Theatre Company, 2002 Dance: Cave's End Choreographer: Rex Nettleford Dancers: David Blake, Marlon Simms, Kevin Moore, Abeldo Gonsales, Mark Phinn, O'Neil Pryce, Germaine Rowe, Patrick Earle & Arsenio Andrade

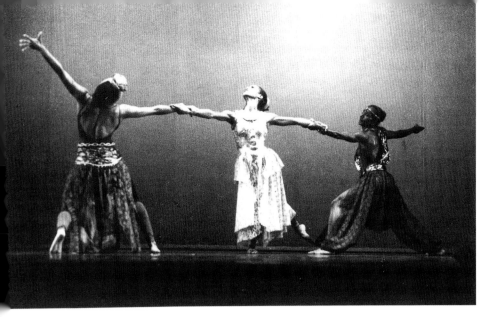

The National Dance Theatre Company, 2002
Dance: Cross Currents
Choreographer: MoniKa Lawrence
Dancers: Natalie Chung, Kerry-Ann Henry &
Carole Orane Andrade

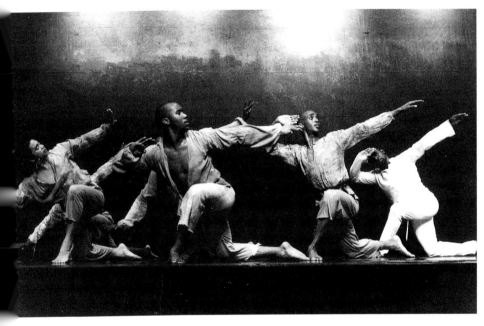

The National Dance Theatre Company, 2002
Dance: The Crossing
Choreographer: Rex Nettleford
Dancers: Abeldo Gonsales, David Blake, Marlon Simms
& Patrick Earle

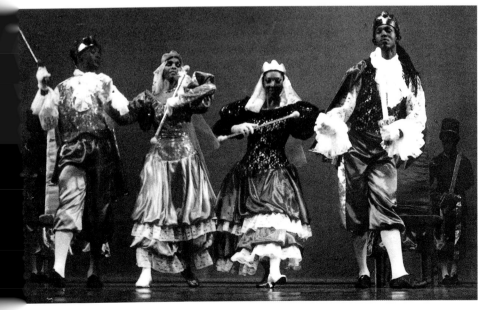

The National Dance Theatre Company, 2002
Dance: Bruckins
Choreographer: Joyce Campbell & Barry Moncrieffe
Dancers: Marlon Simms, Arlene Richards, Alison Symes
& Christopher Walker

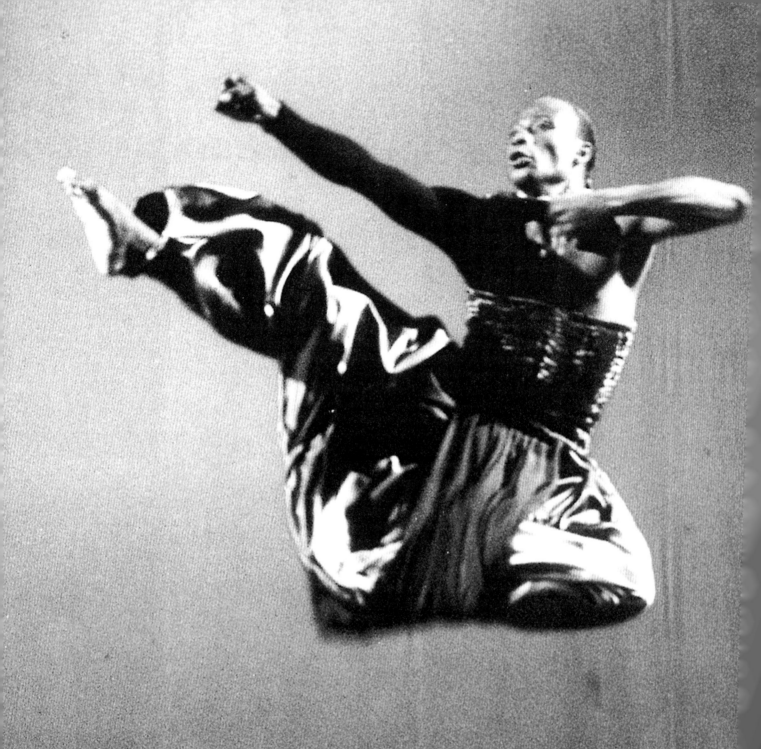

The National Dance Theatre Company, 2002
Dance: Michezo
Choreographer: Tony Wilson
Dancer: Deroi Rose

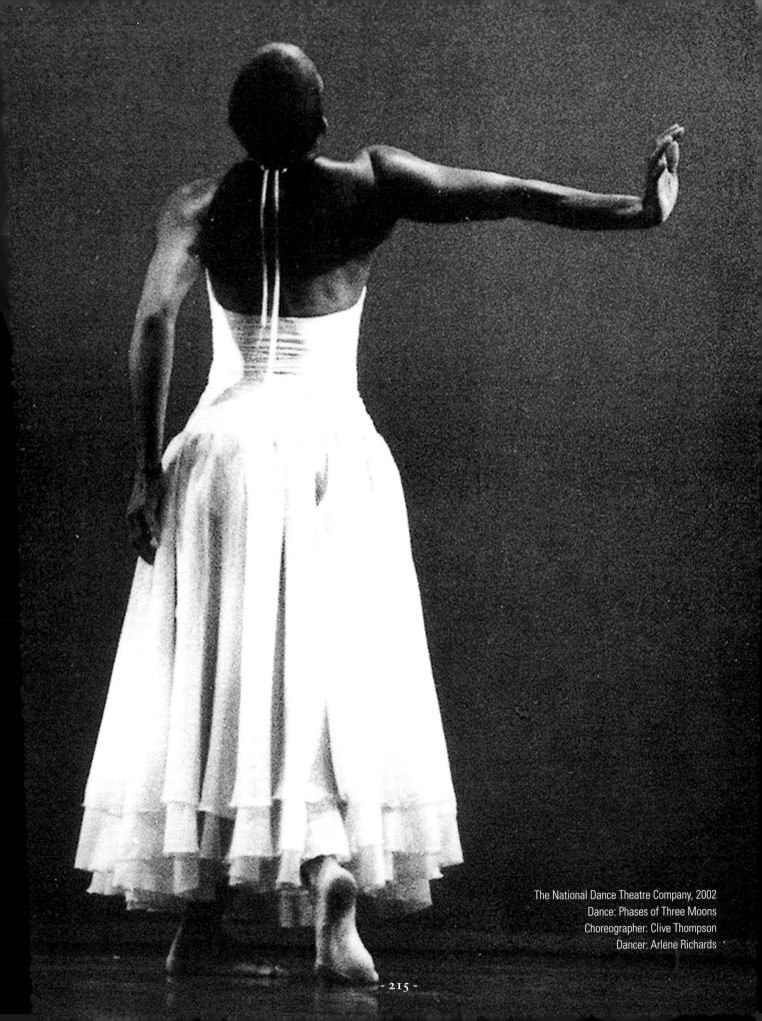

The National Dance Theatre Company, 2002
Dance: Phases of Three Moons
Choreographer: Clive Thompson
Dancer: Arlene Richards

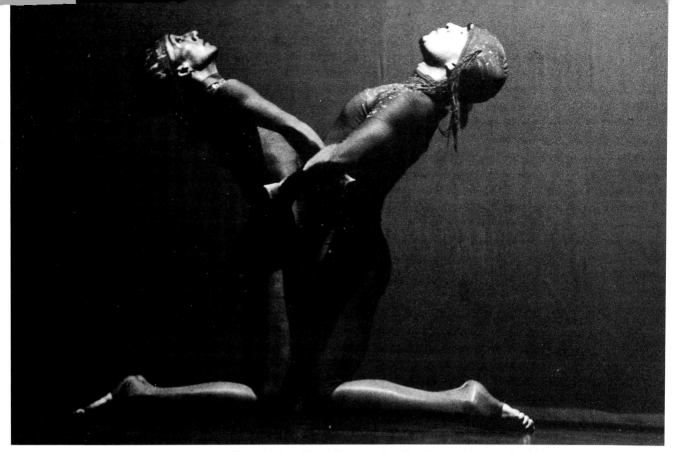

The National Dance Theatre Company, 2002 Dance: **Phases of Three Moons** Choreographer: Clive Thompson Dancers: Carole Orane Andrade & Arsenio Andrade

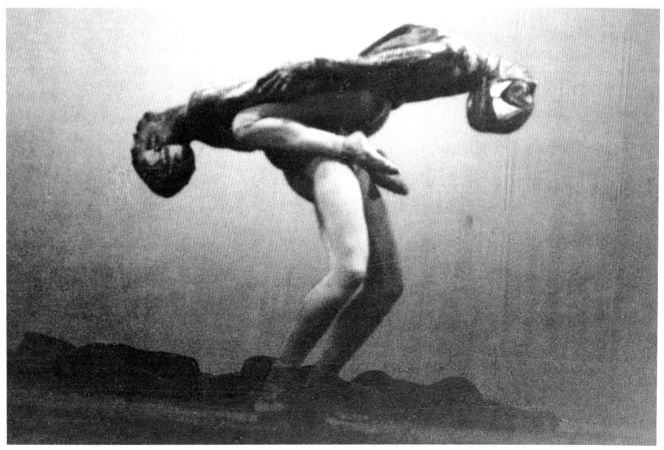

The National Dance Theatre Company, 2002 Dance: **Cocoon** Choreographer: Arlene Richards Dancers: Christopher Walker & Carole Orane Andrade

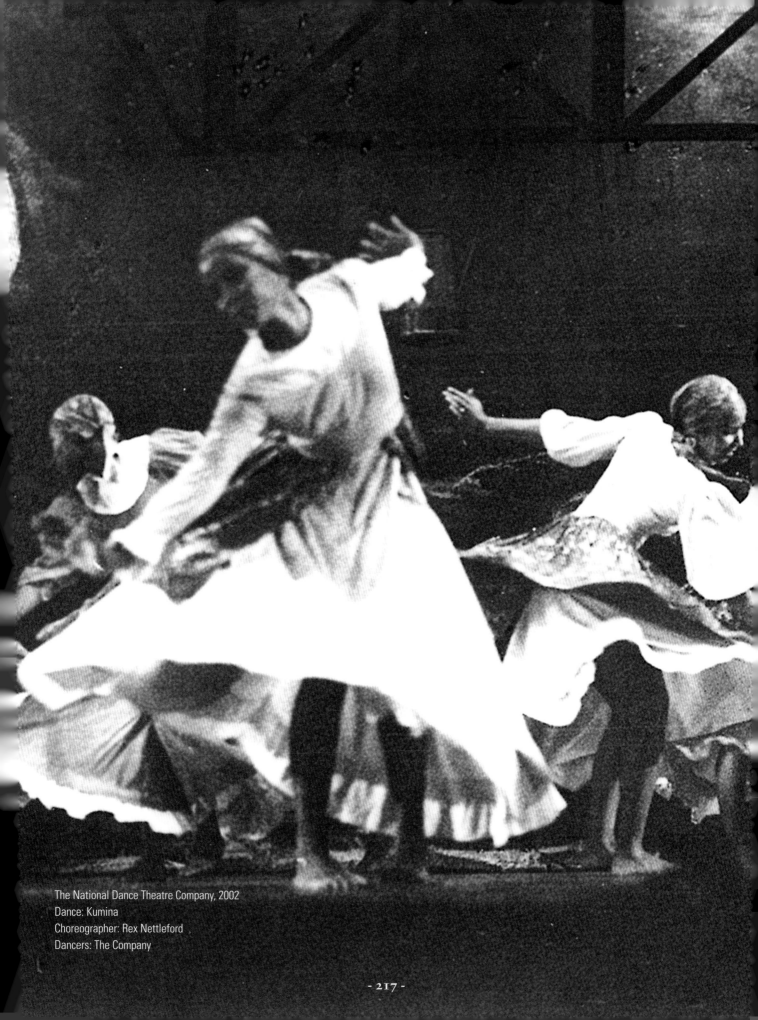

The National Dance Theatre Company, 2002
Dance: Kumina
Choreographer: Rex Nettleford
Dancers: The Company

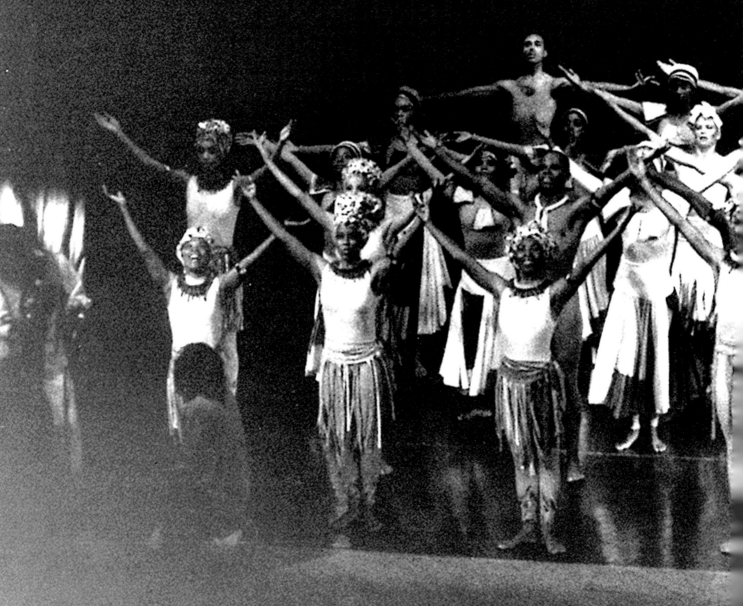

Curtain Call 1993 (Ward Theatre)
Dance: Finale
Dancers: The National Dance Theatre Company, Movements Dance Company,
L'Acadco & The Company Dance Theatre

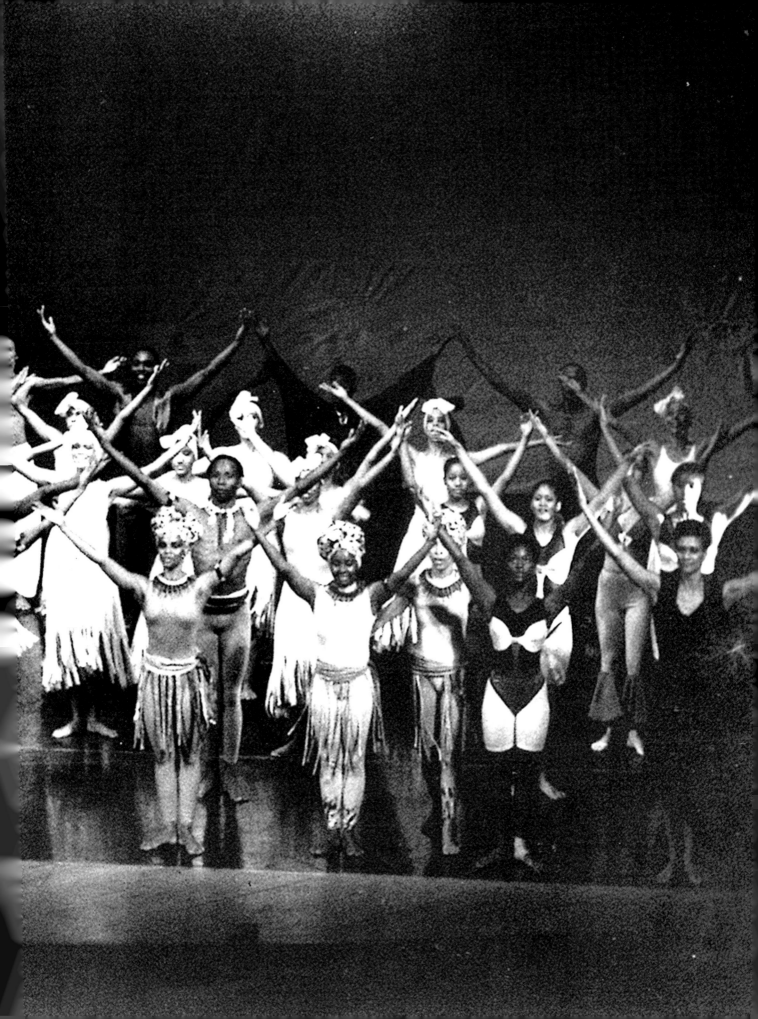

Synopsis of dances

Adagio for Strings, Organ and Six Dancers (1982) This dance is a semi-classical work. It highlights the bond of friendship between five women and the comfort and support provided to one of their number who breaks away and experiences a fleeting relationship with a man. Music: Adagio in G Minor for Strings and Organ by Albinoni Giazotto   *Pages 5, 6*

Alpha (1992) An abstract, modern piece reflecting the beginnings in the womb. The foetus (of no particular sex) seeks its way out. This is a statement of birth and evolution. Music: Vangelis, John Carpenter and Allan Howarth   *Pages 106, 107, 108, 109*

Amathagazelo (1992) A celebration of the African movement. Music: Ashe Lethe Mbuli, Soundtrack of 'Roots', 'Wuzungelum' written by Moongeli Ngema, Becobe, Kupanglogo High Life Music of Ishana Sinda, Traditional Zulu Rhythm from Zulu Land   *Pages 107, 114, 115*

Autumn Breeze (1995) A pas de deux from the ballet 'The Quiet Storm'. Music: Will Downing and Rachelle Ferrell   *Page 49*

Avia Egyptus (1985, 1986) Highly-stylised reggae technique performed on pointe. Music: Cedric Brooks   *Pages 80, 81, 83, 88*

Baka Beyond (1997) Like a flowing river, dance accumulates, integrates, transforms and re-emerges. Music: Martin Cradick and Paddy, LeMercier, and Jerry Goldsmith   *Pages 150, 153*

Belle Caribe (1986)   *Page 71*

Bida Floral (1998) The life force: that man may live… Music: Peter Gabriel   *Page 153*

Bingi (1989, 1990) Nyabinghi rhythms and movements. A spiritual celebration dedicated to a musician who inspired all musicians – Count Ossie. Music: Arranged by Karl Messado (Bingi)   *Pages 91, 100, 102*

Blood Canticles (1996, 2002) Song of Praise, Canticles of Hope, Gifts from the Gods, All in the Blood… Music: Michael Pluznik (Drummer Journey) – 'Above the Starts' Menehune Garden, Johann Sebastian Bach ('Jesu Joy of Man's Desiring'), Marjorie Whylie (Variation of Revival/Poco theme), Abdullah Ibrahim and Johnny Dyani ('Zike'), Dollar Brand – Abdullah Ibraham ('Blues for a Hip King'), Lama Gyourme and Jean Philippe Rykiel ('Souhaits Pour L'Eviel')   *Pages 180, 182, 183, 186, 187, 188, 189, 190, 202*

Brazilian Ode (2002) A suite of dancers inspired by Inaicyra of dos Santos and some ancestral chants and the cult of masculine ancestors (egungun). Music: Iya o Bogunde, Iya Bafete (from Okan Awa sung by Inaicyra); A morte do Capoeira, Sao Bento Grande, Cavalaria (from Capoeira, Cardao de Ouro arranged by Mestre Suassuna e Dirceu); Alabe, Sese Kurundu (sung by Inaicura)   *Pages 203, 212*

Bridges (1983)   *Pages 7, 8*

Bruckins (2002) Music: Traditional arrangement by Marjorie Whylie   *Pages 206, 213*

Bujurama (1996) Of conscious lyrics and …! A celebration of grounded spirituality! Music: Buju Banton (Selections: 'Untold Story' and 'It's not an Easy Road'), Champion (with arrangements by Marjorie Whylie)   *Page 185*

Cave's End (2002) Journey of a lifetime…A light at the end tunnel. Always… Dedicated to Jimmy Cliff for this vision of hope-in-despair. Music: Jimmy Cliff (selections from 'Journeys of a Lifetime' with South Africa traditional Ulwamkelo Iweirokneli (Prologue). Selections are: 'Journeys of a Lifetime', 'Street Vibes', 'Burden Bearer', 'Looking Forward', 'Change'   *Pages 202, 212*

Cease 'N' Settle (1989) Exploring the ethos of the Dance Hall, a phenomenon in Jamaican music and entertainment; a place to 'hold yuh corner' and forget the pressure of ghetto life. Music: Red Dragon, Earle Black, Flouragon and Sanchez, Pinchers, Barrington Levy and the Heptones   *Page 32*

Celebrations (1985) A celebration of Caribbean life utilising dance-forms and other elements of indigenous lifestyles – the love of professionals, a tinge of carnival, the pride of Rastafari, the wit of the Caribbean coquette, the vigour of ritual. Music: Traditional, arranged by Marjorie Whylie   *Pages 170, 171*

Ceremony (1989, 1991, 1994, 1995) An evocation of a rainforest; hunters become animals, the hunted…and oh! the snake goddess   *Pages 31, 32, 33, 36, 46, 51, 52, 53, 54*

Children of Sisyphus (1994) Life has its inherent course and gives its own inherent meaning…and so, even in its most abysmal conditions, man has to continue his struggle to endure… Music: 'Children of the Streets' and 'I Need' by Fr Richard Ho Lung, 'Poor Me Israelite' by Desmond Decker, 'Could It Be Love' by the Wailers Band, 'Running Away', 'Rastaman Chant' and 'Keep On Moving' by Bob Marley, 'Pepper Seed Version' and 'Big Things' by Daddy Screw, 'Big Yellow Taxi' by Monti Alexander, 'Scores' by Wigmore Francis, 'Find Your Way' by Lovindeer, 'Yerri Me' and 'Wat a Wonderful Ting' by the Jamaican Folk Singers, and 'Pocomania' by the NDTC Singers   *Pages 140, 141, 142, 143*

Chosen (2002) It's a trilogy of faith, love and hope. It is dedicated to all who have lost their lives or suffered through violence, terror…lack of love. Music: Dead Can Dance and Mr Cheeks   *Page 63*

Circa 2002 (1996)   *Pages 75, 76*

Cocoon (2002) The Universe – all that is – vast, varied, yet to be explored. What if…? Would you…? Music: Richard Burma, David Arkenstone, Patrick O'Henry   *Pages 209, 216*

Collage (1987)   *Pages 73, 74, 75*

Colours (1994) A swirl of colours inspired by writings, the artistic vision of focus in movement and the influence of an array of music and ideas provided by Rachael Manley's 'A Light Left On'; Susan Alexander's paintings and the sustaining encouragement and support of Glynne Manley. Music: John Dawkworth / Yanni / Excerpts from 'Dead Can'   *Pages 133,134*

Congo Layé (2002) Eulogy to my ancestors, to my blood, to my motherland Africa-Iboya ibo ibo cheche. Music: Conjunto Ballet, Folkloric Afrocubano

Consensus (1993) Myself, the dancers, the Company, as a shared mutual vision of our path to the future   *Pages 131,132*

Cosmic Beat (1994, 1995, 1996) The beat of the drum spoke to every facet of life of our ancestors; its rhythm and spirit the source of a peculiar enduring and powerful energy. That's why 'dem cyaan stop de dance'. Music: Grub Cooper – Africa, Retentions/Echoes and Synthesis Handel Tucker, Maureen Sheridan, Sly Dunbar – Cyaan stop de dance – featuring Junior Reid, Papa San, Carlene Davis, Wayne Wonder, Buju Banton, Junior Tucker, Tony Rebel, Ibo Cooper, Little Lenny, General Degree, Bunny Rugs, Cat Coore, Orville Woods, Jack Radics, Harry T and Sky Juice…   *Pages 45, 56*

Cross Currents (2002) Exploration of the travails of apartheid seen through the eyes of three women of different social castes in South Africa. 'For nothing is more precious in life than a people truly free'. Music: 'Isidawaba singu Fakati' (Lette Mabula), 'Getting into the Habit' (Sister Act), 'Makoti' (Amampondo), 'Carry On' (Latte Mbula)   *Pages 209, 213*

Cry of the Spirit (1996, 1997, 2002) 'Amazing grace, how sweet the sound that saved a wretch like me' – a solo. Music: 'Amazing Grace' sung by Sandi Patti   *Pages 185, 196, 208*

Crystal Jungle (1993) Dance begins in the spirit. Play the drums and the spirit dances. Music: Samite of the Yuganda, Abaana Bakesa: 'Ngabala'   *Page 116*

Dance Jallof (1996) Music: Traditional drum patterns of Ndeup, and Sikyi-Duet Baaba Maal   *Pages 147, 148*

Degagé (1992, 1993) A tribute in dance to nature and flora. Music: Arranged by Calvin Mitchell   *Pages 111, 117*

Dinah's Song (1984, 1986) A recreation of the main theme of Orlando Patterson's novel 'Children of Sisyphus' – to most ghetto dwellers escape is impossible. It traces one woman's struggle to escape and the social forces, which militates against success; even in death she has no release. The initial statement of the ballet highlights the underlying theme – man's existence in the ghetto is no more than that of other denizens – dogs, rats and crows   *Pages 15, 19, 20, 21*

Down to You (1990) Music: Joni Mitchell   *Pages 100, 101, 103, 105*

Dream on Squatters' Mountain (1984) A peaceful village is disturbed by enforcers of the law. The enforcers hunt for victims by harassing all the households each with its worldly possession of a blanket. They conjure up ancestral spirits to fight the evil force and have the enforcers menaced into submission and defeated. After falling asleep exhausted, the wife/mother wakes up, reassured. It was a DREAM… Music: Selections form the score for the South African play 'Poppy Nougena' composed by Sophie Mgcina. Additional music by Nana Vasconcelos-Oridas (Naohios de Petzouila)   *Pages 164, 165, 168*

Drumscore (1996, 2002) When God created the Earth; he first created the drummer (Ghanaian proverb). Music: Caribbean traditional rhythms, melodies arranged by Marjorie Whylie. Sung by the NDTC singers   *Pages 181, 206*

Earth Crisis (1996) We create the world in which we live, continually taking advantage of the Earth's richest offering in order to advance to a 'better' world. Rich is it? Music: Jan Hemmer, Brent Lewis, Vangelis, David Arkenstone (courtest Kirk Waldemar)   *Pages 185. 187*

Echings (1991) Mannequins in a shop window, each having a character. In the silhouette of the after-dark, a little imagination can bring them to life. Music: Duke Ellington   *Page 36*

Echoes (2002) Depicting the balance of nature in the animal kingdom, evolving into the growth of humankind. Women bond, showing their strength of character…the labour of man…and intra-gender relationships that lead to population explosion. Music: Brendan Perry and Lisa Gerrard, Caissons,

Miriam Makeba, Olatunji, Ysaye Barnwell, and Barawen Notes   *Pages 156, 157*

Edna M (1986)   *Page 197*

Elements (1986, 1989) The celebration of Earth, wind, fire and water. Music: Concerts for Sitar by Ravi Shankar, Andre Previn, Mickey Hart / John Williams   *Pages 86, 94, 97*

Elevation (1999) The theme of this dance is centred around the celebrations of the past, where at festival time the family would go to the national stadium to watch the dancing effigies and celebrate. In this dance we try to recapture the lost art of mockajumbie, the art of stilt walking.   *Page 119*

Encounters (1984) An interpretation of George Gershwin's jazz symphony 'Rhapsody in Blue' in celebration of Diaspora Classicism. Music: George Gershwin's 'Rhapsody in Blue' played by the Duke Ellington Orchestra.   *Pages 165, 166*

Evolutia (1986) Man's methods and frustration in searching for individual wisdom – the elements of education, experience and spirituality. Music: Don Cherry 'Rappin Recipe'   *Page 87*

Flashback (1993, 1994, 1995) John is dying. He's all alone and reflecting on his life. He was married but still had to have those occasional flings…plenty of liquor, music and nuff girls. Nobody thought about AIDS because the fun was strictly heterosexual. But somebody was HIV positive and passed the virus on to John. AIDS is everybody's business. Music: Grub Cooper   *Pages 37, 44, 47*

Flashback 'Fear' (2002) A dance depicting fear. Music: Les Baxter 'The Passions'   *Page 203*

Flashback 'Street People' (2002)   *Page 203*

Footprints (2001)   *Page 201*

Forever You (1982, 1986) Duet dedicated to a friend. Music: Barbra Streisand – 'Evergreen'   *Pages 4, 7, 23*

Four Ambiguous Dances (1984) An abstract piece reminiscent in part of a medieval court dance. It is done in four movements: a quintet, solo, duet and trio. Music: Domenico Cimarosa   *Page 15*

Freedom (1996) Music: Dionne Farris   *Page 146*

Fusion (2002) Where cultures meet. Music: Grub Cooper

Genesis (1984, 1986, 1987) It is based on the biblical story of the fall from grace of Adam and Eve. It comprises four sections flowing one into the next – the innocents, knowledge, the intruder and expulsion. Music: Adapted from Gustav Mahler's 5th Symphony   *Pages 10, 11, 12, 13, 18, 25*

Gerrehbenta (1984) The dance takes its name from two of the major traditional rites practiced in Jamaica – 'gerrali' in Hanover and 'dinki-mini' which uses the musical instrument, the benta, in St Mary. Music: Traditional, arranged by Marjoire Whylie. Sung by the NDTC Singers, with Billy Lawrence and Leaford McFarlane (as benta players)   *Pages 162, 163, 169*

Have You Ever Been There? (1985, 1989) Three women among the many insane who roamed Kingston's streets provide the inspiration for the dramatic work. The piece depicts three distinct cases of delusional mental illness. Music: Tchaikovsky: 'Chocolate', version of the Nutcracker Suite   *Pages 85, 91, 96*

He Watcheth (1996) His eyes are always on us, watching our every move, hoping that we become peaceful in his name. Music: 'Eye on the Sparrow' from 'Sister Act II'   *Page 183*

High (1985, 1986, 1992) Set to the driving rhythms of jazz legend Dizzy Gillespie, this piece exposes characters involved in the drug sub-culture of modern society. Music: Dizzy Gillespie – 'Krush'   *Pages 83, 84, 87, 90, 112, 113*

Hold Fast (2001)' *Page 200*

Horizon (1998) When we are at one with God we can be at one with ourselves and can be at peace with each other. Hail the power of the One for in him there is hope. Music: Word/Luciano, Jackie Mitoo, Antoinette Wilson (poem), John O Kee, Zambian Acapella, Everton Blender, Kirk Franklin and Family *Pages 61, 62*

Hounfor of the Drum (1999) A dance giving respect to the trees, animals and the spiritual essence of the oldest musical instrument of man – the drum. Musical Arrangement: Ras Happa *Page 118*

Huapango (1986) A Mexican folklore ballet performed on pointe. Music: Carlos Moncayo 'Huapango' *Page 89*

Images (1989) *Pages 196, 197*

Incantation (2002) The cries of women rupture the fabric between the known and the unknown, creating an interdimensional reality where lamination, hopelessness, regrets and dreams combine, in a confrontation between ancestral forces and contemporary ritual. Music: Toto Bissainthe, Martha Jean Claude, Zao *Pages 204, 205*

Interconnections (1993) Of cross-fertilisation and the sources of energy in the process. Music: Handel's 'Hallelujah Chorus' from 'Messiah' (a soulful celebration); Ba Ba Maal; 'Danibe' from Lain Toro; Miriam Makeba/Nelson Lee 'Welele' and 'Limampondo' from 'Welele'; Mbongeni Ngema 'The Lord's Prayer' from 'Sarafina' (The Sound of Freedom); Dorothy Musaka 'Kuthenizulu' from 'Pata Pata'Huapango (1986) A Mexican folklore ballet performed on pointe. Music: Carlos Moncayo 'Huapango' *Page 174*

Interlude (1988) A love duet. Music: Barbra Streisand *Page 29*

Islands (1985) This includes: i) Homecoming; ii) Rite of Passage; iii) Worksong; iv) Paradise; v) Paradise Lost; vi) Lament; vii) Islands; viii) Coral coquette; ix) Carnival. Music: Irving Burgie and traditional, arranged and conducted by Larry Ashurore and played by the Royal Philharmonic Orchestra, London *Page 169*

Jamboree (1986) This is a folk work, which highlights the flavour and nuances of Caribbean dance forms. Music: Caribbean Drum Rhythms and Ralph Mac-Donald *Page 20*

Kumina (1996, 2002) This is based on the Jamaican Afro-cult, to be found largely in St Thomas. The rites are held for a variety of occasions – for mourning, tombing, healing, thanksgiving and even when help is needed to win a court case or for winning a lover. Music: Traditional, with James Walker (Playing cast) and the NDTC drummers and singers *Page 184, 206, 217*

Lament (1986, 1990) Reminiscences of a relationship. Music: Al Benezie 'Leyenda' *Page 105*

Legacy of the Duke (2002) Visions and movements evoked by the sounds of Duke Ellington. A celebration… Music: Duke Ellington *Page 211*

Libertad (1992) Walk, run, cry, scream – fight for freedom. Music: Brian and Tony Gold's 'Can You', 'Sweet Honey on the Rock' *Page 112*

Life Cycle (1985) The united functioning of body organs to support an instrument called the human body, and reaction of that instrument to infection and disease. Music: Penguin Café Orchestra *Page 85*

Lilac Blossom (1987) A dance in tribute to the late Edna Manley: etchings of an artist, mother and stateswoman. Music: Hubert Lawes *Page 24*

Liza (1998) Based on the folk song of a young girl who likes to gossip, this dance explores the character Liza…and unearths a warm-hearted country girl who is full of zest for life and its potential, but who is also bored with the tranquillity of rural life. She gives in to the attraction of the bright lights of the city and finds love, but is overcome by the rapid pace of the city. She migrates yet again, but this time to the life she knows – life in the country. Music: 'Linstead Market' and 'DJ Chant' by Maurice Gordon, 'Liza' sung by Chrissie D and arranged by Danny Brownie, 'Mout a Massie' sung by Chrissie D, Patsy Ricketts and Gabrielle Harban, 'Country Life' by Wigmore Francis: Shaggy *Page 153*

Llow Mi Nuh (1986, 1990) A look at oppression in its various forms. Music: A collage of reggae music and speeches by Malcolm X and U Thant *Pages 86, 99, 101*

Lotus Flower (1993) A three-part ballet, which looks at the natural revolution of the Earth. In ancient Egypt folklore, land surrounding a fertile valley was burned by the Sun, reducing the valley into a small desert oasis. Mother Egypt Flower, mother of all lotus flowers is strong in faith and will. Though she ultimately succumbs, she holds steadfast against the killer Sun long enough so that the roots beneath her are saved for future generations. Music: Soliman Jamil *Page 41*

Love Games (1986) *Page 72*

Love Joy (1993) Dedicated to the memory of the late Ivy Baxter, pioneer of Jamaica's modern dance movement. 'The Spirit of Remembrance is eternal'. Music: Finesse and Billy Joel *Page 41*

Magic Movements (1987) A love duet. Music: Crystal Gayle – 'A Long and Lasting Love' *Page 25*

Many Rivers to Cross (1990) A pas de deux from 'Tribute to Cliff' which shows the invincibility of the human spirit and to Jimmy Cliff's ever-present sense of hope. Music: Jimmy Cliff *Page 104*

Mayur (1995) The theme of the dance is the feeling of joy and happiness felt by the peacock when the dark clouds appear on the horizon to herald the onset of the rainy season in India. Music: Traditional *Page 174*

Michezo (2002) Music: Papa Wemba, Drums from Uganda, Mickey Hart, Bad Boys from Brazi *Pages 202, 214*

Millenial Beings (2002) *Page 207*

Missioner (1988) A reflection on the life of Alexander Bedward, religious leader, folk hero, faith healer and certified lunatic, whose failure to ascend to heaven caused his followers to lose hope. Music: Sweet Honey in the Rock, Bach, Billy Lawrence and Anthony Wilson; Poem/Prologue: Easton Lee *Page 28*

Mitosis (1985) This dance symbolises the phases of cell division or 'Mitosis' – the essence of life. Music: Soundtrack from the movie 'Young Lovers' / Heaven and Hell *Page 17*

Moments (1997) Three different women…three different spaces…with pleasant memories. Music: Bob Marley, Antonio Banderas with Madonna and Enigma *Pages 148, 149, 156*

Morpheus Webb (1997) 'Was it a vision, or a waking dream? Do I wake or sleep?' (John Keats) Music: The Taliesin Orchestra – Enya *Page 151*

Next (1985) A hilarious presentation of a Reggae Broadway audition. Music: Taj Mahal: 'When I feel the Sea beneath My Feet', Marvin Gaye: 'Third World Girl' *Page 84*

No Frills (1997) No story… no messages… just fun! Music: Ewan Simpson, and O'Neil Mundle *Page 152*

Noisy Art (1990) A witty interpretation on the mechanisms of a clock. Music: Various artists   *Page 103*

Oshumare (Rainbow) (1995, 1996) A dance which celebrates the influences of Africa on modern dance theatre – the sprinkling of spirit and form. Music: Ju Experience (Nigerian Afro jazz musicians) edited by Grub Cooper with the finale by Grub Cooper   *Pages 49, 55, 57*

Outamany (1985) Music: Various Jamaican artists   *Page 82*

Part of My Soul (1987, 1988) A tribute to Nelson and Winnie Mandela: their love, their inspiration to the struggle against apartheid and the fight to free Nelson. Music: Miriam and Hugh Makeba   *Pages 26, 27*

Pepperpot (2002) A blend of Jamaica's cultural dance forms that have been highly influenced by our African heritage – ranging from deep traditional Kumina and Pukkumina to contemporary urban Nyabingh. Music: NDTC singers, and the Mystic Revelation of Rastafari   *Page 157*

Phases (1986)   *Page 73*

Phases of Three Moons (2002) From the boundless deep, the moon arises wondrous. Glorifying the evening like a beauteous maiden. Now she adorns herself in unconscious duty. Eager, anxious that we recognise her beauty… (for Sonia Jones). Music: Hector Villa-Lobos, Charles Ives   *Pages 210, 215, 216*

Pressure (1984, 1985, 1986, 1989, 1995) This work explores yet another dimension of reggae music: dub poetry. It attempts to capture Oku Onuora's constant focus on the pressure and hardships facing poor people and the intensity of the poet himself. It also attempts to reflect through dance, and the strength of the male dancer in particular, the raging mood and concerns of this poet. Music: Oku Onuora   *Pages 11, 13, 14, 16, 17, 18, 30, 50, 55*

Prisms (1994) A refraction, a reflection of power, the beauty, the passion that are within. Music: Mickey Hart / John Williams   *Page 135*

Puncie (1985) An urban romp: Some boys are playing dominoes on the sidewalk. Puncie, fresh from the country, is preparing to go out on the town with her yard-friends. The sight of her disrupts the game among the boys. The sight of the boys goads her into innocent flirtation. She ends up attracting all of them. Music: Peter Ashbourne: Suite for his Jamaica – Story of Jamaica   *Page 173*

Rah (1995) 'The journey continues…And in a thousand years still she will rise. She is the source of life. Her radiance inspires, her power compels, she can be cruel, but she is…Hurrah.' Music: Various; additional music (finale) by Steve Golding and Arlene Richards   *Page 179*

Recollections (1984) 'I've loved you all my lives before, and now I'll let you know. The dreams I've dreamed in death… silence… they grow… Our love… is endless' (C. Thompson) Music: Ramsay Lewis   *Pages 168, 169*

Red City (1992) Various aspects of city life are portrayed – the good, the bad and the ugly. All that glitters is not gold   *Pages 124, 125, 126, 127*

Reminiscence (1984) A love solo. Music: 'All I want from You' sung by Nina Simone   *Page 167*

Rhythm Branches (1993) A celebration of roots and rhythm. Music: Ultramarine and Grub Cooper   *Page 37*

Rose Hall (1993) A very striking and curious story founded in fact, it is set in nineteenth century Jamaica and surrounds the Rose Hall Sugar Estate owned by Annie Palmer, known and feared among her slaves as the 'White Witch'. Music: 'Carmina Burana' by Karl Orff, 'Ghost' soundtrack by Maurice Jarre (excerpts), 'Dracula' soundtrack by Wojciech Kilar (excerpts), 'Back to the Future' soundtrack by Alan Silvestri (excerpts). Selected recordings by: Enigma, Enya, Sting, Wagner, Depeche Mode, Hermeto, David Rudder, Strunz & Farah, Dave Grusin   *Pages 127, 128, 129,130*

Ruth (1983) Ruth, a Maobite woman, loses her husband Mahlon, an Israelite. She shows unusual loyalty to her mother-in-law, Naomi, and follows her to Bethlehem at the beginning of the harvest season. There she meets Boaz, a wealthy citizen, marries him and becomes the ancestress of the Messiah. Music: Jean Sebelius, Tchaikovsky, Ester and Carl Orff   *Page 8*

Sacred Ground (2001)   *Pages 201, 205*

Satta (1986, 1989, 1993) The several qualities of primordial women are glorified in this sensuous tribute – which draws its movement theme from the Egypto-Yoruba Oricha (gods) dances   *Pages 88, 90, 93, 94, 96, 98, 116*

Selah (1997) 'Everyone wants to go to heaven. Nobody wants to die'. Amen. Music: Marjorie Whylie and sung by the NDTC Singers with soloist Vin James: Alleluia Amen, Chant of the Spirits – by Marjorie Whylie: The Holy City by Stephen Adams, Lord God of Abraham from Elijah by Mendelssohn: The Beckoning Trumpet by Marjorie Whylie – trumpet soloist, Leighton Johnson, Yanni   *Page 195*

Serenade (1986) A montage of our historical past: in recognition of Jamaica's National Motto 'Out of many One People'. Music: Pre-Hispanic music of Mexico, Josef Zawinoc and Steel Pulse   *Page 22*

Shades (1989) Music and dance; differentiation and synthesis. Music: David Sanborn, Mango Santamaria   *Page 30*

Shades (1990) Music: Hugh Dawes   *Page 104*

Side By Side (1998) For my sisters. Hopes and dreams, joys and fears; happiness, sadness, gladness… shared. A special bond that lasts forever. Music: 'Art of Noise', Vangelis   *Page 198*

Silent Partner (1989) A dancer, her space and her faithful companion…the Barre. Music: A medley of evocative music from Glen Miller and Flora Purim   *Page 94*

Snake Pit (1996) Experience the Moment. Music: Carmina Burana, and Jerry Goldsmith   *Page 145, 146*

Space (1997) When you dream, you can do anything you want …Reality is different. Music: Robert Clivilles, and Rene Dupere   *Page 151*

Spirits at a Gathering (1995, 1998) Of sister-friendships; brother-bondings and the healing acceptance of differences. Of love, of faith and mutual caring – all in a life which is our 'Gathering'. Music: 'Deep Forest' by Mouquest/Sanchez; Dan Lacksingh (producer)   *Pages 175, 179, 199*

Steal Away (1997)   *Pages 191, 192, 194*

Sulkari (1985) A dance of exaltation of fecundity and fertility, so that through the man/woman relationship human life will continue. The focus of the dance was inspired by and originates from the sculpture, carvings, headdresses, masks, stools and other elements and details of African sculpture, as well as the movement of the Yoruba peoples of Amara (Dahoney). Music: Traditional Afro-Cuba (Yoruba) collected and arranged by Eduardo Rivera. Adapted by Marjorie Whylie and sung by the NDTC Singers   *Page 172*

Syncrisis (1989) A comparison of opposites, costumed dramatically in black and white. Music: 'Walking in your